RENAL DIET COOKBOOK

The Complete Renal Diet Book to Get Your Life Back With Easy Recipes

(Renal Recipes to Increase Your Kidney Health)

Vance Perlman

Published by Alex Howard

© **Vance Perlman**

All Rights Reserved

Renal Diet Cookbook: The Complete Renal Diet Book to Get Your Life Back
With Easy Recipes (Renal Recipes to Increase Your Kidney Health)

ISBN 978-1-989891-89-6

Legal & Disclaimer

The information contained in this book is not designed to replace or take the place of any form of medicine or professional medical advice. The information in this book has been provided for educational and entertainment purposes only.

TABLE OF CONTENTS

Part 1

Introduction

Chronic kidney disease (CKD) is a major public health problem. A systematic review, based on population studies from developed countries, described an average prevalence of 7.2% (individuals over 30 years old). According to EPIRCE study data, it affects approximately 10% of the Spanish adult population and more than 20% of people over 60 years of age, and it is surely underdiagnosed. In patients followed in Primary Care with diseases as frequent as arterial hypertension (AHT) or diabetes mellitus (DM), the prevalence of CKD can reach 35-40%. The magnitude of the problem is even greater, considering the increase in morbidity and mortality, especially cardiovascular, related to renal impairment.

CKD is considered the final common destination for a constellation of pathologies that affect the kidney chronically and irreversibly. Once the diagnostic and therapeutic measures of primary kidney disease have been exhausted, CKD involves common and generally independent protocols for action.

The most frequent causes of ERCA with their corresponding links are described in this ebook. Often more than one cause co-exist and enhance kidney damage.

- Diabetic nephropathy
- Arteriosclerotic vascular disease, nephroangiosclerosis, ischemic nephropathy. Concepts all that have in common the presence of arterial hypertension.
- Primary or secondary glomerular disease to systemic disease
- Congenital and hereditary nephropathies
- Interstitial nephropathies
- Prolonged obstruction of the urinary tract (including lithiasis)
- Urinary tract infections
- Systemic diseases (lupus, vasculitis, myeloma, etc.)

In this chapter, we will review the clinical aspects and conservative management of CKD. Diagnoses and treatments of specific renal diseases are discussed in the corresponding chapters, and nutrition needed to counter the diseases with different recipes.

Chapter 1

Definition And Stages

CKD in adults is defined as the presence of a renal structural or functional alteration (sediment, image, histology) that persists for more than 3 months, with or without deterioration of renal function; or a glomerular filtration rate (GFR) <60 ml / min / 1.73 m2 without other signs of kidney disease. The KDIGO guidelines have introduced renal transplant patients, regardless of the degree of renal failure they present. Markers of renal damage are considered:

- Elevated proteinuria
- Alterations in the urinary sediment
- Electrolyte abnormalities or other alterations of tubular origin
- Histological structural alterations
- Structural alterations in imaging tests

The severity of CKD has been classified into five categories or grades, depending on the GFR and three categories of albuminuria. This is because proteinuria stands out as the most potent modifiable prognostic factor for CKD progression. The deterioration of GFR is a characteristic of grades 3-5, the presence of other signs of kidney damage not being necessary. However, in categories 1 and 2, the presence of other signs of kidney damage is required. This is a dynamic classification and usually in constant revision. This classification, which undergoes slight subtle changes over time, has the advantage of unifying language when referring to the definition and magnitude of the problem, previously defined as CKD. Therefore, the methodology for the measurement of GFR and the determination of proteinuria are critical tools for the diagnosis and management of CKD.

Glomerular filtration measurement

The GFR is a critical parameter for the staging of CKD, its management, and monitoring.

Direct markers (inulin, DTPA, EDTA, iothalamate, iohexol) are more accurate than creatinine clearance (KCR), but their complicated methodology makes them unfeasible in routine clinical practice.

The KCr is the most comprehensive test, but when the FG drops, the tubular creatinine secretion (Cr) increases, so it overestimates the real FG by 10-30%. It also entails the potential error in the 24-hour collection.

The normal range of serum Cr is 0.8-1.3 mg/dl in men and 0.6-1.0 mg/dl in women. Changes of ± 0.3 mg/dl in different laboratories may be considered intercensal changes. Cr begins to increase when the FG drops 50%. In advanced phases, small changes in GFR cause a significant increase in serum Cr.

Formulas have been developed for the calculation of GFR from serum Cr along with analytical, demographic, and anthropometric variables, obviating the need to collect 24-hour urine. Currently, the most used in research and clinical practice are the MDRD in its simplified format (4 variables) or complete (6 variables) and the CKD-EPI (Chronic Kidney Disease Epidemiology Collaboration) equation, which has shown better results regarding accuracy and precision. The Cockcroft equation is less accurate in patients older than 65 years or with extreme weights.

The website of the Spanish Society of Nephrology provides the most common equations for the calculation of the GFR.

Additionally, such as the use of cimetidine, semisuma of KCr, and Kurea or cystatin are not applied in daily practice, and its use has been reduced.

Finally, although it is desirable to improve methodological accuracy, periodic monitoring of serum Cr is useful to know if the GFR changes or remains stable.

- **Proteinuria**

The magnitude of proteinuria is the main modifiable factor that decisively influences the prognosis and clinical decision-making, being also an independent factor of cardiovascular risk. It has a direct renal toxic effect, induces inflammation and tubulointerstitial fibrosis, and contributes to the loss of nephron mass.

The Spanish Society of Nephrology has published a Consensus Document for the assessment of proteinuria in renal patients. Briefly, 24-hour urine collection is considered the gold standard, but it is difficult to guarantee the complete selection. The simultaneous determination of Cr in the urine sample allows establishing the albumin ratio of total protein / Cr, which has a good correlation with the elimination in 24 hours. In both adults and children, we recommend the determination of this ratio in an isolated urine sample.

The albumin excretion range that extends between 30 and 300 mg/ 24 hours (20-200 ug/min) is classically known as microalbuminuria, being more recently replaced by "moderately elevated albuminuria." These limits include the range from the upper level of normal urinary excretion to the level of unequivocal detectability of proteinuria detection strips. This range of persistent albuminuria for> 3 months is a risk factor for progressive renal deterioration, as well as adverse cardiovascular events. It should be considered a manifestation of diffuse endothelial damage, being an indication of renoprotective practices and modification of cardiovascular risk factors. In any case, albuminuria should be considered as such in the absence of factors that may increase it circumstantially, such as urinary infections, physical exercise, fever, or heart failure.

Population screening with test strips is indicated only in patients who are at risk of CKD. If the proteinuria is harmful or only traces, it determines the albumin/creatinine ratio in an isolated urine sample. If positive, the protein/creatinine ratio in the urine sample should be calculated, as well as a renal diagnostic evaluation must be indicated.

In CKD, these ranges do not help since monitoring of patients with higher proteinuria from more than 300 mg/day, up to 6-8g/day, and even being a continuous variable, cut-off points should be established in predicting the risk better. Proteinuria and albuminuria can be considered equivalent in high ranges (> 1500 mg/d). In the range between 300 and 1500, there may be significant differences.

Glomerular hyperfiltration

Within the pathophysiological mechanisms involved in the development and progression of CKD, glomerular hyperfiltration has been the object of intense study since Brenner B described it in 1996. The pathological increase in GF would explain the progression of renal insufficiency and glomerular structural damage in patients with a reduced number of functioning nephrons. Experimental data have shown that states with reduced renal mass lead to glomerular sclerosis of functioning nephrons. Hyper protein diets can accelerate this phenomenon. The reduction in the number of nephrons causes hyperfiltration in intact nephrons, with a decrease in resistance in afferent and efferent arterioles (less in these), glomerular and increased flow, and GFR. This results in functional and structural changes in the endothelium, epithelium, and mesangial cells, which causes micro thrombosis, microaneurysms, expansion of the glomerular mesangium, and subsequent glomerular sclerosis. Obesity and diabetes are hyperfiltration situations with average renal mass.

Chapter 2

Risk Factor

Numerous risk factors for the onset and progression of CKD have been described, which, in turn, can enhance the effect of primary kidney disease if this is the case. Although most of these factors have shown more association than causation, often inconsistency, simultaneous co-existence is frequent and enhances the damage. Several have common pathophysiological mechanisms, with proteinuria and glomerular hyperfiltration being the most prevalent and vital:

- Non-modifiable conditions: age, sex, race, and low birth weight.
- Comorbid alterations potentially modifiable, and that directly or indirectly can induce renal damage: HT, diabetes, obesity, dyslipidemia, smoking, hyperuricemia, hypoalbuminemia, and cardiovascular disease.
- Alterations are inherent to CKD and that have been proposed as risk factors for progression: anemia, changes in mineral metabolism, metabolic acidosis. Its handling is discussed in the corresponding sections.
- Other molecules have also been described and associated with progression of renal damage, such as asymmetric dimethylarginine (ADMA) or FGF23, among others without to date, having relevance in the clinical scenario, or there is any recommendation.

Non-modifiable risk factors

- **Age**

Advanced age is a well-known risk factor for CKD. However, it is not a factor of progression in itself, beyond the natural functional impairment associated with age ("old kidney"). In our experience, advanced age appears paradoxically as a protective factor, but two circumstances limit this statement: 1) the patient's exit competes with the arrival to dialysis in the multivariate analysis, and 2) elderly patients who arrive at ERCA consultations are less proteinuric. When adjusted for proteinuria, the apparent protection of advanced kidney disease to develop terminal kidney disease disappeared.

Debate on the "kidney of the old": the decrease in GFR - as well as the increase in proteinuria - represent a disease, or is it the natural result of aging? It is assumed that according to changes in renal hemodynamics with aging, approximately one ml/mn/year is lost after 40 years. With aging, glomerular sclerosis, tubular atrophy, and vascular sclerosis are noted. But there are also elderly individuals in whom the expected decrease infiltration is not observed.

- **Male sex**

Described in population studies as an independent prognostic factor of suffering from CKD, but has not been verified by other authors. However, in all records of renal patients, male sex represents approximately 60% of patients undergoing renal replacement therapy. It is not clear as a factor of progression in itself; there were several circumstances associated with sex that are determining factors in the evolution of renal damage.

- **Black or African American race**

In the USA, a higher incidence in dialysis of the African-American population is demonstrated. This circumstance should be attributed mainly to the higher prevalence of severe HT, worse sociocultural conditions, and possibly genetic factors.

- **Low birth weight**

Low birth weight is associated with a small number of nephrons and subsequent development of CKD. The acquired loss of renal mass, experimental or clinical is associated with glomerular hypertension and hyperfiltration.

- **Sociocultural deprivation**

Epidemiological studies demonstrate that low social, cultural, and economic levels are associated with worse health. Kidney disease does not escape these circumstances.

- **Modifiable Risk Factors**

Although the factors indicated below are predictors of onset and progression of CKD, all directly or indirectly are subordinated to the magnitude of proteinuria. This being the most significant risk factor for progression. Hence, the management of CKD is based primarily on antiproteinuric measures.

- **Hta**

Associated mostly with CKD, more than 75% of patients suffer from it. It is both the cause and consequence of CKD.

In general, clinical blood pressure figures <140/90 mmHg are recommended in patients with CKD. However, this objective can be reduced to 130/80 mmHg in diabetic or proteinuria patients. In patients with AHT and CKD, especially if they have diabetes, ambulatory blood pressure monitoring (ABPM) is recommended, given the frequency of masked hypertension, or nightly increase in blood pressure. Ambulatory Blood Pressure Measurement. What Is the International Consensus?

- **Diabetes**

It is a potent initiating factor, being the most frequent cause of terminal CKD. In ERCA consultations, its prevalence can currently reach 40-50% of patients. As a factor of progression, proteinuria conditioned by diabetic nephropathy is the main predictor. The degree of progression depends directly on the magnitude of the proteinuria: diabetics and non-diabetics progress the same to similar levels of proteinuria.

Also, in population studies, elevated HbA1 levels have been associated with an increased risk of CKD. The control of diabetes should be a priority, especially in protein patients.

- **Obesity**

Overweight and obesity are increasingly frequent in patients with CKD (See nutritional changes in CKD) as a reflection of what happens in the general population, being also the prelude to diabetes. Population studies have shown a strong association between obesity and the risk of CKD. Excess weight is associated with glomerular hyperfiltration. Besides the risk of renal impairment, they generate an additional problem to include a patient on the transplant waiting list. That is why nutritional measures combined with appropriate physical exercise are mandatory in these patients.

- **Dyslipidemia**

It is well known that dyslipidemia hurts the vascular tree in general. In CKD, there is a high prevalence of dyslipidemia, and there is experimental evidence that it adversely influences the progression of renal damage, although it has not been verified in controlled clinical studies. In any case, the evaluation and therapeutic intervention for the control of dyslipidemia in the renal patient are mandatory.

- **Smoking**

Smoking is a recognized cardiovascular risk factor and is proposed as an independent renal risk factor, although its mechanisms are not established. It should be considered one of the essential remediable risk factors. So, tobacco withdrawal is a priority recommendation in CKD.

- **Hyperuricemia**

Hyperuricemia (See Uric acid and chronic kidney disease) is considered when its serum values are> 7 mg/dl. It can be asymptomatic or cause diseases such as uric nephrolithiasis, uric acid nephropathy, tophaceous gout, acute gouty arthritis, and asymptomatic hyperuricemia.

In CKD, several factors can increase uric acid levels: Use of diuretics increased vascular, renal resistance, or coexistence of insulin resistance.

Patients with CKD frequently have hyperuricemia associated with the fall of GFR, which in most cases, is asymptomatic. Hyperuricemia has been associated with an increased risk of cardiovascular morbidity and mortality, hypertension, development of nephropathy in diabetic patients, and although not fully verified, the progression of CKD. These are sufficient reasons to systematically treat elevated uric acid levels, even in asymptomatic patients. Besides, this is not recognized in all consensus documents.

Risk Factors Inherent In Chronic Kidney Disease

Anemia and alterations of mineral metabolism - and within these more specifically hyperphosphatemia - have been associated with more rapid renal deterioration. However, these factors are a consequence of kidney damage, so it is difficult to isolate their effect as predictors. In any case, the correction of anemia and mineral metabolism alterations are indicated from early ERC phrases.

Metabolic acidosis is common in CKD due to poor elimination of acid load by the kidney. It has also been described as an unfavorable factor in the progression of CKD and should be prevented and adequately treated.

Chapter 3 Diagnosis For Chronic Kidney Disease

The general precepts of the practice of internal medicine should be applied. The diagnosis of acute renal failure and its differential criteria are addressed in the corresponding section.

Clinic history

Particular attention should be given to urinary symptoms, such as nocturia, polyuria, polydipsia, dysuria, or hematuria. A complete history of systemic diseases, exposure to renal toxins, infections, and possible family history of kidney disease must also be obtained.

Physical exploration

Weight, height, and possible malformations and developmental disorders should be recorded. It is important to take blood pressure, the examination of the fundus, examination of the cardiovascular system and chest, and abdominal palpation looking for palpable masses, or kidneys with lumbar contact. In men, a rectal examination is essential to examine the prostate. Signs of edema can be seen on the extremities, and the state of peripheral pulses must be explored.

Biochemical parameters

Urinalysis: hematuria, proteinuria, cylinders (blood cylinders), and evaluation of renal function. Alterations associated with CKD: anemia, mineral metabolism (Ca, P, PTH), and acid-base balance.

Ultrasound Imaging diagnosis

Mandatory tests in all cases must be carried out to first verify that there are two kidneys, measure their size, analyze their morphology, and rule out urinary obstruction.

Small kidneys (below 9 cm, depending on the body surface) indicate chronicity and irreversibility. Normal-sized kidneys favor the diagnosis of an acute process. However, polycystic kidney disease, amyloidosis, or diabetes can occur with healthy or enlarged kidneys.

If the kidneys have a size difference greater than 2 cm, this may be due to pathology of the renal artery, vesicoureteral reflux, or varying degrees of unilateral renal hypoplasia.

- **Eco-doppler**

It is the first renal imaging scan in any patient. Inexperienced hands are the first diagnostic step of uni or bilateral renal artery stenosis.

Duplex Doppler: It has the advantage of providing anatomical and functional data of the renal arteries. Direct visualization of the renal artery (mode B) is combined with the measurement (doppler) of blood flow and its characteristics.

- **Intravenous urography**

Not indicated for the diagnosis of CKD since it provides limited information because no contrast is eliminated. This being also nephrotoxic, being able to precipitate entry into dialysis. It has been fallen into disuse with ultrasound benefits.

- **Digital angiography**

The gold standard for the diagnosis of renal vascular diseases is arteriography, but it has the disadvantage of contrast toxicity.

The first examination at this time in any patient is the performance of a doppler, and later, if the renal function is normal, a CT angiography or a magnetic antiresonance can be indicated, according to the experience of each center.

Angio-CT or helical Scanner: Its most significant advantage is the administration of intravenous contrast, which gives room to visualize the caliber of the light and the characteristics of the arterial wall in three dimensions. Its limitation is contrast toxicity in a patient with renal impairment.

Magnetic antiresonance: It is an increasingly used technique in patients with normal renal function and not recommended in patients with grade 3-4 renal insufficiency, given the gadolinium toxicity (See Nephrogenic systemic fibrosis).

Angiography with CO_2 obviates contrast toxicity, but the risk of atheroembolic disease in patients with peripheral artery disease must be kept in mind.

Modern techniques of antiresonance with image intensification offer excellent information about the vascular tree without using gadolinium.

Renal biopsy

It is an invasive and risk-free procedure, indicated when there are diagnostic doubts of primary kidney disease or a high degree of chronicity of tissue damage. We must assess their possible risks against the potential benefits of the information you can provide. If done in the early stages of the ERC, your information may be useful. In advanced stages, we will often encounter sclerosed and terminal kidneys.

Chapter 4: A Diet For Chronic Kidney Disease

The chronic kidney disease (CKD) refers to the continuous deterioration of the kidneys that progress over time (You can learn more about the relationship between IRC CKD here). It is clinically detected when the glomerular filtration rate (GFR) falls below 60ml/min for at least three months, but it is not until it drops below 30ml / min that marked symptomatology occurs.

"Once the CRI has been detected, the diet becomes an unmatched strategy to help prevent or slow the deterioration of the kidneys, which is why what we eat and drink becomes important."

The recommendations of the diet of the person with CRF will vary depending on the stage and the characteristics of the disease itself, but they must take the following parameters into account:

Control of protein intake: A restriction of dietary proteins should be made because the substances derived from their metabolism (urea, creatine, and phosphates) accelerate the evolution of the disease.

Sodium intake control: In renal failure, the kidneys are not able to remove excess sodium to maintain the body's balance. Also, sodium intervenes in our blood pressure and favors fluid retention, as well as causing a more excellent sensation of thirst, which can compromise fluid intake.

Control of potassium intake: Potassium is an essential mineral to maintain healthy nerve and muscle function. In renal insufficiency, the kidney is unable to eliminate the potassium that we ingest, being able to produce, if it accumulates in excess, muscular weakness, cramps, and even compromise our heart rate.

Phosphorus intake: Phosphorus is a mineral present in all foods, although in varying amounts. In renal failure, it accumulates in the blood and is responsible for vascular calcification and progressive deterioration of the bones.

Among these parameters, according to the state of the pathology, fluid intake should also be taken into consideration. So, this intake should be adapted to the hydration and the diuresis state of the person, or the nephrologist will determine the volume of fluid that can be ingested.

One of the most common risks of this protein-restricted diet is malnutrition, which we must ensure adequate caloric intake. To do this, consider the contribution of carbohydrates (the main component of food such as rice or fruit) that corresponds will prove to be a good option. In this case, take them in their refined version (for example, in flour, pasta, etc.) since the integral versions have high amounts of minerals, especially phosphorus. With the same purpose, lipids (usually called 'fats' are the main component of foods, such as oil, butter, sauces such as mayonnaise, etc.). They also provide us with calories, helping to enrich our diet, but it's necessary to choose those rich in unsaturated fats (such as olive oil).

To facilitate that the intake of minerals with involvement in the pathology corresponds to the indicated restriction, it's essential to know their content in foods, as well as their recommended consumption frequencies. Also, to reduce this mineral content of the foods to be consumed, we must follow some recommendations on their cooking techniques. These culinary tips and recommendations will facilitate the elimination of a part of this mineral content so that the intake will be even lower.

For an adequate establishment of this food planning, the reading of nutritional labels will be critical, since they are usually a complete source of information that helps in choosing the most suitable foods. Likewise, we must attend to the concept of ration since it will be necessary to adjust the ratios of some food groups with particular attention to proteins, and thus, not compromise health.

Chapter 5: Steps To Control Chronic Kidney Failure

Seek treatment for hypertension

The pressure is now considered the leading cause of chronic renal failure. According to nephrologist Nestor Scho, professor at Unifesp, the increase in blood pressure damages the blood vessels of the kidney and may cause hypertensive nephropathy. "This way, the organ becomes overloaded, and little by little loses its filtering capacity," he explains. Taking care of hypertension is essential even when it is not the cause of chronic renal failure as it becomes even more important in the advanced stage of the disease.

Control of diabetes

"Diabetes is the second leading cause of chronic renal failure," says nephrologist Lucio Roberto Requião Moura of Hospital Israelita Albert Einstein. This is because the disease triggers the so-called diabetic nephropathy, a change in kidney vessels that leads to a protein loss in the urine. Also, diabetes favors atherosclerosis – the formation of plaque fat in the arteries that hinders the filtration work of the kidneys. Over time, more and more toxic substances are trapped in the body, which can lead to death. One way to detect the problem, therefore, is to do urine tests to find out if the protein is being eliminated or not. Those already diagnosed with diabetes need to be more aware of their kidney health.

Watch the weight

Overweight people (Discover their ideal weight) have a higher risk of developing hypertension and diabetes, which is reason enough not to let the scale hand rise, says nephrologist Lucio.

Also, obesity alters the way blood reaches the kidneys by the influence of certain hormones, overloading the organ. Moreso, being overweight is a risk factor for high cholesterol and triglycerides.

Adapt your diet

When it comes to food, analyzing the underlying disease that triggered kidney failure is critical. If it is diabetes, for example, the diet should be the right diet for those with diabetes. If it is hypertension, then there should be reduced salt intake. "However, in general, it is recommended that the patient avoid excessive protein intake, especially of animal origin, which gives rise to toxic elements in the body that would make the kidneys work harder," explains nephrologist Nestor. In specific cases of insufficiency yet, there may be retention of potassium in the body. Patients with this problem need to prepare food in a way that causes them to release some of this nutrient. Vegetables, for example, need to be cooked.

Inquire about medications

The self-medication is dangerous even for healthy people. For those with kidney failure, however, self-medication without proper medical evaluation can accelerate kidney deterioration. "The most dangerous are non-hormonal anti-inflammatory drugs," warns nephrologist Lucio. Therefore, explain your problem at the beginning of every medical appointment to avoid aggravating the disease.

Way to drink alcohol

Although no studies are proving the isolated relationship between alcohol intake and chronic renal failure, alcohol abuse compromises the functioning of the body as a whole. Thus, it is recommended to handle consumption. If you are having a drink, however, nephrologist Nestor advises opting for wine. "It contains antioxidants that can help eliminate concentrated toxins in the body.

Put out the cigarette.

"Cigarettes are responsible for worsening blood pressure levels, and are still involved with hormonal changes that worsen kidney function," explains nephrologist Lucio. Also, smoking triggers a vasoconstriction effect, decreasing the volume of blood filtered by the kidneys. In this case, there is no moderation option. The patient must end the addiction.

Practice exercises

The last recommended care for chronic kidney failure sufferers is regular exercise. "It prevents diabetes, hypertension, obesity, among other problems, and improves circulation and kidney function," says nephrologist Nestor. According to him, any activity is already better than physical inactivity, but it is always recommended to seek training that pleases the patient so that he does not feel discouraged over time.

Chapter 6: Importance Of Exercise With Kidney Disease

The United States is the country where more research studies are conducted on physical activity and kidney disease. A survey of the United States Kidney Data System (USRDS) and studies on Dialysis, Morbidity, and Mortality showed that 35% of 2264 patients on dialysis indicated that they did not perform any leisure-time physical activity, and only 50% did exercise more than once a week. Some authors believe that people with CKD experience a deterioration of bodily function, which is another restriction for the development of the physical activity. Research has shown that an increase in physical activity levels reduces the onset of fatigue and improves physical function levels.

In another study, in the United States, 37% of 99 patients undergoing hemodialysis did not exercise regularly. In this study, they also consider the number of patients and the activities they performed. In general, these patients were spending 4.5 hours per week in all exercise, such as work or household tasks, which relates to leisure. This meager amount of activities can explain, in part, why these patients had proven to be significantly less active than even the general sedentary population when the activity was objectified with accelerometry (system to quantify the physical activity that a person performs throughout of the day).

REPETITION

CKD patients, especially dialysis patients, suffer marked muscle loss and excessive fatigue. It is known that inactivity, muscular atrophy, and reduced physical function are associated with increased mortality in CKD. Known causes include uremic myopathy, neuropathy, inactivity, and anemia. Exercise in patients receiving dialysis treatment was introduced first three decades ago, but it is a treatment offered in a few renal units worldwide despite the scientific evidence supporting its application.

Is It Necessary To Exercise?

WHY?

Physical activity is associated with the improvement of the level of health of the general population and patients with renal insufficiency.

The Centers for Disease Control and the American College of Sports Medicine (ACSM) recommend that all adults exercise for, at least, 30 minutes every day. There are many reasons to encourage physical activity in the general population. Among them, we can highlight the improvement of general health, the reduction in the number of hospitalizations, and the improvement of the quality of life related to health. Since it has been shown that physical activity decreases cardiovascular risk factors in the general population, it is worth asking whether the benefit of physical activity can also be transferred to patients with chronic kidney disease (CKD), who are a population of high cardiovascular risk. The answer is, "YES."

It is necessary to work to increase awareness of the potential benefits of a higher level of physical activity for patients with CKD. One of the most natural causes of population growth with kidney disease is derived from a sedentary lifestyle, which translates into an increase in morbidity and mortality. Patients with CKD, who receive hemodialysis (HD) and peritoneal dialysis (PD) have a considerable decrease in exercise tolerance, functional capacity, and endurance and strength, as well as less muscle mass than healthy subjects, or which patients with severe chronic renal failure who still do not need renal replacement therapy.

To improve the quality of life of patients undergoing dialysis or transplantation, exercise programs planned and supervised by professionals should be included in their rehabilitation. There are many studies in the scientific literature on physical training in patients with CKD in HD referred to the health-related physical condition. In contrast, the research regarding the physical health of transplant patients on peritoneal dialysis is scarce.

Chapter 7: Renal Diet Recipes

Liver of heifer and its onion compote

INGREDIENTS

- 1 slice of organic heifer liver
- 2 small onions
- 1 apple Canada
- tablespoon olive oil
- 1 lemon
- 1 slice of cinnamon
- Salt pepper

DIRECTIONS

1. Peel and slice the onions. Make them return in half of the olive oil until they become translucent. Salt and pepper them. Cover and cook on very low heat for 30 minutes. Watch for cooking, add a little water if necessary.
2. Wash the lemon under running water, wipe and squeeze it.
3. Wash the apple, peel it, and remove the fibrous core and seeds. Cut it into cubes. Lemon it to avoid blackening, then place in a small saucepan with cinnamon and add 2 tablespoons of water. Cook covered over low heat for 20 minutes. At the end of cooking, crush it in the coarse compote.
4. Cut the liver into strips and cook for 2 to 3 minutes in the pan with the remaining olive oil. Once cooked, mix it with the onion compote.
5. Enjoy it immediately, accompanied by the applesauce.

Nutritional interest

Thanks to the liver, this dish is very rich in iron and zinc, and it is easily assimilated. Also, trace elements essential for the proper functioning of the immune system. It may be recommended particularly for young children, regulated women, and endurance athletes, who often lack iron.

In case of excess cholesterol, do not consume more than one shot per week.

Palette of pork and its vegetables

INGREDIENTS

- 1 pallet of bone-in pork of 1 kilo
- 100g smoked diced bacon
- 1/4 green cabbage
- 300g carrots
- 200g turnips
- 400g of firm-fleshed potatoes type BF 15
- 2 onions
- 2 cloves
- 1 bouquet garni
- 1 tablet of organic vegetable broth
- Salt pepper

DIRECTIONS

1. Place the bacon in a saute pan and sauté over medium heat, stirring. Add the palette and use the fat rendered to brown the meat, about 5 minutes on each side. Add a peeled onion and chopped, also brown. Add 1/2 liter of water, the bouquet garni, and the second onion stuck cloves and the crumbled broth.
2. Wash the piece of cabbage, remove the hard outer leaves and its core. Dip it in a pan of boiling salted water and let it whiten for 10 minutes. Drain and cut it into strips. Add it to

the sauté pan with the palette, salt, and pepper it. Then continue cooking for 15 minutes.
3. Wash and peel carrots, turnips, and potatoes. Cut them into slices. Add the carrots and turnips in the pan, then add salt and pepper. Continue cooking for 10 minutes. Add the potatoes and finish cooking for 20 minutes. Rectify the seasoning, and remove the bouquet garni and onion pique clove.

Nutritional interest

This complete dish simultaneously brings functional meat proteins, fiber, and vitamins from vegetables, energy carbohydrates from potatoes. Low fat, it is suitable for overweight (450 kcal per serving). For a balanced meal, add milk and seasonal fruit.

Exotic Fruit Verrines

INGREDIENTS

- 2 kiwis
- 1 mango
- 1/2 grenade
- 1/4 liter of semi-skimmed milk
- 2 eggs
- 25g of sugar
- 1 vanilla pod
- 2 half-sheets of gelatin or 1/2 teaspoon of agar agar
-

DIRECTION

1. Wash the vanilla pod, slice it in half, and place it in a saucepan with the milk. Heat and stop the fire just before boiling. Let the vanilla steep in the milk.
2. Position the gelatin in a bowl of water (cold).

3. Separate the whites and egg yolks. Whip the yolks with the sugar. Add the cooled and filtered milk. Pour everything into the saucepan and cook on low heat, then constantly stir until the cream thickens. Add drained half-leaves of gelatin or agar-agar, wait for their complete dissolution to cut the fire. Divide the custard into four glasses and refrigerate for at least 2 hours.
4. Wash the fruits under running water and sponge them out. Peel the kiwis and mango and cut them into cubes. Collect the grains from the pomegranate. Mix these fruits gently and divide them into the glasses. Enjoy it immediately.

Nutritional interest

Thanks to exotic fruits, these verrines are rich in antioxidant vitamins: beta-carotene, vitamins B9, and C, which defends the body against infections.

To balance your menu, consume a verrine at the end of a meal with vegetables, meat, fish or legumes, and starchy foods.

Chickpea Salad

INGREDIENTS

- 150g chickpeas
- 1 onion
- 1 clove
- 1 clove of garlic
- 1 bouquet garni
- 200 g celery-branch
- 1 lemon
- 5 tablespoons of olive oil
- 1 tip of curry
- 1 tablespoon chopped chives
- Salt pepper

DIRECTION

1. Position the chickpeas in a large bowl filled with cold water and let them soak for 12 hours.
2. Peel the onion and garlic. Drain the chickpeas. Place them in a casserole with 1/2 liter of cold water, the bouquet garni, and the onion stuck clove, the clove of garlic, some grains of pepper. Cover, cook for 2 hours.
3. Wash the celery, detach its branches from the bulb, remove the top of the leaves, detail it in the sticks.
4. Wash the lemon and squeeze its juice — mix two tablespoons with the olive oil and the curry.
5. Drain the chickpeas well. Mix with celery. Add salt and pepper. Season with the olive oil vinaigrette and add the chives.

Nutritional interest

- This salad, rich in fiber and protein (chickpeas) is very satiating and has a low glycemic index. It can be especially recommended in case of diabetes. Calorie intake reasonable 250 kcal per serving. It is suitable for overweight.
- The consumption of pulses is recommended, at least twice a week, to increase vegetable protein and reduce animal protein.

Roquefort pear toast

INGREDIENTS

- 8 slices of walnut bread (120g)
- 1 jar of 100g of white cheese with 3% fat
- 60g of Roquefort cheese
- 2 ripe Williams or Guyot pears
- 1 lemon

- 4 nuts

DIRECTIONS

1. Toast the slices of bread.
2. Remove the nuts from their shells.
3. Mix the cottage cheese and Roquefort cheese. Spread toast with this mixture.
4. Wash the lemon, sponge it, and squeeze its juice.
5. Wash the pears, peel them, remove their central part and their pips, divide them into tiny dice. Lemon immediately to prevent the pears from turning black.
6. Spread the pears over the toasts. Add a walnut kernel per toast.

Nutritional interest

- Made from walnut bread, Roquefort pear toasts provide 25% of the recommended daily intake of omega 3 essential fats, which are beneficial for cardiovascular prevention. They are rich in fiber (bread, pear, nuts), satiating, and regulating the transit.
- Spread with lean fresh cheese with 3% fat and a small amount of Roquefort. They are suitable for hypercholesterolemia.
- Whether you eat them as a starter or as an appetizer, you can balance your meal by moderating starchy foods and preparing vegetables.

Shortbread with jam

INGREDIENTS

- 100g of wheat flour type 55
- 50g butter or margarine rich in omega 3 not lightened
- 50g of sugar

- 1 egg
- 120g of strawberry or apricot jam, homemade if possible
- 2 tablespoons icing sugar
- 1 large star-shaped cookie cutter
- 1 round-shaped cookie cutter 1.5 cm in diameter

DIRECTIONS

1. Separate the whites from the egg yolk.
2. In a bowl, mix the flour, sugar, and butter until you have a texture of sand. Add the egg yolk to mix the dough ball. Let the dough rest in the refrigerator for at least 30 minutes.
3. Preheat the oven to 180 ° C. Arrange a sheet of baking paper on a baking sheet.
4. Spread the dough. Cut star-shaped shortbread. In half of these shortbreads, cut a small circle of dough in the middle.
5. Arrange the shortbread on the plate and bake for 15 minutes.
6. Let the shortbread a little cool. Cover each shortbread with jam and sprinkle each shortbread with icing sugar. Arrange the shortbreads pierced over jammed biscuits.

Nutritional interest

- Made with flour and jam. These biscuits are rich in carbohydrates and energy. They have their place at the end of a meal without starch or snack after a light lunch. They can also be used as a snack or in recovery after a sports training.
- Low in fat, they are suitable for hypercholesterolemia.

Skewers of seitan

INGREDIENTS

- 1 block of seitan 240g
- 1 lemon

- 3 tablespoons sesame oil
- 2 onions
- 1 clove of garlic
- 1 tablespoon acacia honey
- 1 tablespoon paprika
- 200g cherry tomatoes
- 100g of Paris mushrooms
- 2 tablespoons sesame seeds
- Salt pepper

DIRECTIONS

1. Wash the lemon under running water, sponge it, and squeeze it.
2. Peel the onions, slice them. Peel and slice the clove of garlic.
3. Cut the seitan into cubes.
4. Mix honey and lemon juice, add oil and paprika, salt, and pepper. Arrange the seitan, onions, and garlic in a dish and sprinkle with the marinade. Allow in the refrigerator for at least 1 hour.
5. Wash the tomatoes and mushrooms, sponge them out. Cut the mushrooms into strips.
6. Make skewers by alternating seitan cubes with onion rings, cherry tomatoes, and mushroom slices. Filter the marinade.
7. Cook the kebabs on a pan in their marinade, 2 min 30 on each side over medium heat. Drain and roll them in the sesame seeds, then iron for 1 min in the pan to lightly brown the sesame seeds.

Nutritional interest

These skewers provide as much protein as a small steak, the quality of which can be optimized by combining legume proteins, such as lentils. With a reasonable energy intake of 280 kcal, they are suitable for overweight.

Bean salad to shell

INGREDIENTS

- 150g of shelling beans
- 30g pasta, farfalle type
- 150g fresh green beans
- 200g tomatoes
- 1 carrot
- 1 bouquet garni
- 4 tablespoons olive oil
- 2 tablespoons balsamic vinegar
- 1/2 teaspoon of mustard
- 1 shallot
- 2 teaspoons chopped parsley
- 1 teaspoon chopped basil
- Salt pepper

DIRECTIONS

1. Shell the beans. Position them in a large saucepan and cover them completely with cold water. Add the bouquet garni, cover the pan. Let it simmer for 35 minutes.
2. Wash the green beans and mop them up. Cut in half, salt, and steam for 15 minutes.
3. Cook the pasta the time indicated on the package.
4. Peel and chop the shallot.
5. Prepare the vinaigrette with oil, vinegar, mustard, salt, and pepper. Add the shallot.
6. Wash tomatoes and carrot under running water. Rind off and grate the carrot, then cut the tomatoes into wedges.
7. In a salad bowl, combine the shelling beans and the drained pasta, the green beans, the tomatoes, the carrot, and the herbs. Add the vinaigrette and mix gently. Correct the seasoning if necessary.

Nutritional interest

This salad is rich in fiber and antioxidants: vitamin E, vitamin C, lycopene (tomatoes), beta-carotene (carrot). It combines the complementary proteins of beans to shelling and pasta. By doubling the proportions, you will get a balanced vegetarian main course.

Raspberry tartlets without gluten

INGREDIENTS

- 100g of rice flour
- 30g of almond powder
- 30g butter or margarine rich in omega 3 not lightened
- 90g of sugar
- 2 eggs
- 20g of cornflower
- 25 cl of semi-skimmed milk
- 1 vanilla pod
- 500g raspberries
- 1 tablespoon icing sugar

DIRECTIONS

1. Heat the milk until boiling. Cut the fire. Split the vanilla pod in half and let it steep in the milk.
2. Mix the rice flour with the almond powder and 60 g sugar. Add the melted butter and work the dough with a fork until you get a sandy texture. Combine the dough with one beaten egg and refrigerate for at least 30 minutes.
3. Separate the white and yellow from the remaining egg. Whip the yolk with 30 g of sugar. Add the cornflower, then the milk, previously filtered, very gradually. Cook this cream over

low heat, constantly stirring until thickened (about 3 minutes).

4. Preheat the oven to 180° C. Spread the pie dough and divide it into four lightly greased tart pans. Cover each tart with parchment paper and dried vegetables — Cook the tarts for 25 minutes.
5. Wash the raspberries under a stream of running water. Sponge them carefully and remove their peduncles.
6. Wait until the tartlets are cold to garnish with pastry cream and raspberries. Sprinkle with icing sugar.

Nutritional interest

Made from rice flour and corn, this tart is suitable for gluten intolerance. Thanks to raspberries, it is a good source of fiber and vitamin C. It's energetic, and has its place at the end of a meal without starchy foods.

Quiche with ratatouille

INGREDIENTS

- 250g of flour
- 125 g butter or margarine rich in omega 3 not lightened
- 2 zucchini
- 1 eggplant
- 3 tomatoes
- 1 yellow pepper
- 1 onion
- 2 tablespoons olive oil
- 1 bouquet garni
- 4 eggs
- 100 g grated Emmental cheese
- Salt pepper

DIRECTIONS

1. In a small salad bowl, mix the flour and butter until you have a texture of sand. Add a little salt water to combine the ball of dough. Let stand in the refrigerator for at least 30 minutes.
2. Peel and slice the onion. Wash the vegetables. Peel the zucchini and cut into slices. Cut the eggplant into cubes. Remove the peduncle, seeds and whitish fibrous parts of pepper, cut into strips.
3. Fry the onion with the olive oil contained in a frying pan. Add pepper, zucchini, and eggplant, brown while stirring. Add the tomatoes, the bouquet garni, salt, and pepper. Cover; simmer on low heat for 20-30 minutes. At the end of cooking, discover to let evaporate the water of constitution of vegetables.
4. Preheat the oven to 200-210 ° C. Spread the dough and place it in a pie dish. Cover with parchment paper and dried vegetables — Cook for 20 minutes.
5. Mix the well-reduced ratatouille with the eggs and Emmental cheese. Pour this mixture onto the pie shell, free of parchment paper. Finish cooking in the oven for 15 minutes.

Nutritional interest

The ratatouille quiche is a complete balanced dish, which can be supplemented with dairy and fresh fruit.

Zucchini/shrimp verrines

INGREDIENTS
- 2 zucchini
- 2 shallots
- 2 tablespoons olive oil
- 1/4 teaspoon of curry
- 100 g shelled shrimp
- 1 bunch of chervil
- Salt pepper

DIRECTION

1. Peel and mince the shallots.
2. Wash the zucchini, sponge them, peel them, and cut them in small dice.
3. Place the oil in a pan with the curry. Add the shallots and zucchini to make them come back. Add salt and pepper. Cover, cook for 15-20 minutes over low heat. At the end of cooking, if necessary, evaporate the vegetable water.
4. Divide the zucchini fondue into 4 verrines. Add the shrimp on top, and decorate with chervil sprigs.

Nutritional interest

Made from ingredients from the Mediterranean diet. This verrine provides multiple antioxidants (vitamins C and E, beta-carotene, polyphenols, and selenium) to protect health. Very low fat and low in calories (100 kcal per serving), it is particularly suitable for hypercholesterolemia or overweight.

Homemade Sauerkraut

INGREDIENTS

- 1 white cabbage, preferably organic
- 2 teaspoons of salt
- 1 teaspoon juniper berries
- 1 teaspoon of peppercorns
- 6 bay leaves
- 2 glass jars of 1 liter with a screw lid

DIRECTION

1. Wash the jars and their lid thoroughly.
2. Put away the outer leaves and the core of the cabbage. Cut it into skinny strips.

3. In each jar, alternate layers of cabbage, each with salt, juniper berries, peppercorns, and bay leaves. Pack well.
4. If there is a bit of room at the top of the jar, add boiled or chilled water. Close the jars without screwing them in completely.
5. Leave the jars at room temperature for 2 days so that the cabbage can ferment. Then, screw them thoroughly and place them in the refrigerator for 1 month before eating. You can keep them for up to 6 months. Once started, consume them within 48 hours.

Nutritional interest

- Preparing homemade sauerkraut helps to consume raw. And so, to enjoy more of its vitamins (C and B9 in particular) and natural lactic ferments at the origin of its obtaining. Some of these ferments reach the colon alive and contribute to the functional diversity of the microbiota (intestinal flora), favorable to health.
- Namely: 100g of sauerkraut provides 100% of the daily need for vitamin K, a contribution that people on anticoagulant therapy must consider.

Homemade Yogurts With A Pressure Cooker

INGREDIENTS

- 90cl of semi-skimmed UHT milk
- 1 jar of plain yogurt with whole commercial milk
- 4 tablespoons of skimmed milk powder
- 1 organic orange
- 1 cooking thermometer

DIRECTIONS

1. Wash the orange under running water, sponge it with absorbent paper and recover its zest.
2. Place the milk and orange zest in a saucepan, heat to a boil. Then, turn off the heat, and let the zest infuse until the milk temperature drops to 45 ° C (check with the thermometer).
3. During this time, fill the pressure cooker with water for one third. Close the lid and put it on the fire. Leave several minutes under pressure. Then, cut the fire and let the steam escape.
4. Sift the milk through the sieve to remove the orange zest. Whisk it with yogurt and milk powder. Divide into eight glass yogurt jars.
5. Discard the boiling water from the pressure cooker. Place the pots in the basket of the casserole and enclose them immediately in the still very hot casserole. Let it ferment at room temperature for 4 - 5 hours. Then place the yogurt in the refrigerator.

Nutritional interest

Yogurt makes it possible to take advantage of the good proteins and the calcium of the milk, even in case of intolerance to lactose (sugar of cow, goat, and sheep milk), that its lactic ferments have the capacity to digest. It can be called probiotic because its regular consumption contributes to the development within the microbiota (intestinal flora) of bacteria considered as beneficial to human health.

Omelet With Chicken Livers

INGREDIENTS

- 6 eggs
- 150g of chicken livers
- 2 shallots

- 3 tablespoons of olive oil
- 1 tsp chopped parsley, 1 teaspoon chopped chives, 1 tsp chopped tarragon
- Salt pepper

DIRECTIONS

1. Pare and cut in 4 the chicken livers. Peel and mince the shallots.
2. Fry the chicken livers in the olive oil and cook for 3 to 4 minutes. Then, reserve and sweat the shallots over a fairly soft fire. Mix them with the livers and reserve.
3. Beat the eggs, add salt, and pepper. Cook them in a sloppy omelet. Spread over the chicken livers and herbs.
4. Fold the omelet and slide it onto a serving dish.

Nutritional interest

- Poultry liver omelet provides good protein that is effective for growing children, as well as maintaining muscle mass in adults. It is a good source of vitamin D: 2g per serving, or 40% of the recommended daily intake.
- Its reasonable caloric intake (225 kcal) allows us to consume it in case of overweight.
- To know: this recipe is not recommended for pregnant women and children under three years because of the very high vitamin A content of chicken livers.

Cheesecake

INGREDIENTS

- 350g of 3% fat (3% fat) white cheese enriched with vitamin D (Calin + type)
- 2 eggs

- 35 g of Maïzena ®
- 60g of sugar
- 1 teaspoon of bitter almond extract
- 1 tablespoon flaked almonds
- Salt

DIRECTIONS

1. Preheat the oven to 170 ° C. Garnish a mold to run out of baking paper.
2. Separate the yolks and whites from the eggs. Climb these in very firm snow with a pinch of salt.
3. Mix the Maïzena® gradually with the cottage cheese. Then add the egg yolks, the sugar, then the almond extract. When the preparation is homogeneous, gently add the egg whites.
4. Pour the dough into the mold and bake for 40 to 45 minutes. Check the cooking by pricking the cake with a knife tip. Wait until it has cooled down to remove the baking paper.
5. Pass the almonds quickly in a non-stick frying pan for browning. Decorate the cake.

Nutritional interest

The cottage cheesecake provides good protein (cottage cheese, egg), as well as energy carbohydrates (sugar, Maizena). Made from white cheese enriched with calcium and vitamin D. It provides respectively 25 and 100% of the recommended daily intake of an adult in these micronutrients. It may be recommended particularly to prevent osteoporosis for growing teenagers and seniors.

Pear And Walnut

INGREDIENTS

- 1 beautiful pear
- 80g of butter
- 1/2 teaspoon of vanilla extract
- 2 eggs
- 100g of sugar
- 50g of chestnut flour
- 50g of wheat flour type 55
- 1/2 sachet of yeast
- 80g unsweetened cocoa powder
- 14 nuts
- 2 teaspoons icing sugar

DIRECTIONS

1. Preheat the oven to 180 - 200 ° C. Lightly grease a non-stick mold with an oiled brush.
2. Wash the pear, peel it, remove its central part and its seeds, and cut it in big quarters. Put it in the pan with 20g of butter and vanilla. Remove it from the fire as soon as it begins to caramelize. Arrange it at the bottom of the mold.
3. Schell nuts.
4. Separate the whites from the egg yolks. Beat the egg whites with a pinch of salt.
5. Mix the egg yolks with the sugar. Add the remaining 60 g of butter. Gradually add the two flours with the yeast, then the cocoa powder, and finally 12 nuts. Carefully incorporate the whites into the snow.
6. Pour the mix into the pan over the pear and bake for 25 minutes at 180° C. Check the cooking with a knife tip (the dough does not stick when the cake is cooked).
7. Unmount the pound. Sprinkle with icing sugar and decorate with the remaining two nuts

Potato salad with smoked herring

INGREDIENTS

- 400 g of firm-fleshed potatoes such as Amandine or Belle de Fontenay
- 1 small beet
- 2 shallots
- 150 g sweet smoked herring fillets
- 4 tablespoons ISIO 4 mixed oil
- 2 tablespoons vinegar
- 1 teaspoon of mustard
- 2 teaspoons chopped dill (fresh or frozen)
- Salt pepper

DIRECTIONS

1. Wash the potatoes under running water, peel them, slice them and steam them for 20 minutes.
2. Cut the herring into cubes.
3. Peel the beetroot and cut into cubes. Peel and slice the shallots
4. Mix mustard, oil, vinegar, and shallots.
5. Divide the still-warm potatoes and beet into 4 serving plates. Salt very lightly and pepper. Add herring and vinaigrette, sprinkle with dill. Taste immediately

Nutritional interest

- This salad is rich in protein (herring), as well as in fiber and complex carbohydrates (potato). But, his main interests are his contributions of essential omega three and vitamin D, abundant in oil ISIO 4 and herring. One serving provides about 12 grams of vitamin D, more than double the recommended daily intake.
- This salad is suitable for diabetes or overweight (250 kcal per person), provided it is consumed within a balanced meal, combined with a tasty vegetable dish, a dairy, and fresh seasonal fruit.

Salmon With Lentils

INGREDIENTS

- 1 salmon steak
- 50g du Puy lentils
- 1 carrot
- 1 onion
- 1 bouquet garni
- 1 small white leek
- 1 teaspoon dried tomatoes
- 1 shallot
- 1 tablespoon olive oil
- 1 tablespoon dry white wine
- Salt and pepper

DIRECTIONS

1. Wash the carrot and peel it. Peel the onion. Cut these vegetables into large slices. Place them with the lentils and the bouquet garni in a saucepan. Cover with cold water, cover, and cook for 30 minutes in small broths. Salt at the end of cooking, remove bouquet garni, and slices of vegetables.
2. Wash the leek and thinly slice it. Peel and chop the shallot. Sweat these vegetables with olive oil. Then add the white wine and 2 tablespoons of water, cover, and then cook on low heat for 20 minutes. Add the dried tomatoes, a little water if necessary, and finish cooking 10 min.
3. Steam the salmon for 10 minutes.
4. Arrange salmon and lentils on a serving platter. Spread over the leek fondue.

Nutritional interest

Very rich in proteins (salmon, lentils) and fiber (lentils, vegetables). This main course is particularly satisfying.

Associated with a dairy and a fruit, it allows us to "hold" without hunger until the next meal and never to nibble. It is particularly suitable for diabetes or overweight (510 kcal per serving).

SPINACH EGG CAKE

INGREDIENTS

- 1 commercial buckwheat pancake
- 150g spinach
- 1 egg
- 1 tablespoon of olive oil
- One teaspoon chopped parsley
- Salt pepper

DIRECTIONS

1. Wash the spinach under running water with a filter. Drain them in a dishcloth or salad spinner. Remove their tail and ribs if necessary. Place in a pan with olive oil, salt, and pepper. Let them cook for 5 minutes on high heat, just until their water evaporates. Reserve them.
2. Place the pancake in the pan so that it warms up. Garnish with spinach. Break the egg over the center, salt, and pepper. As soon as the white is cooked, remove the pan from the heat.
3. Sprinkle with parsley and fold the four corners of the cake. Enjoy it immediately.

Nutritional interest

- The egg whip spinach is a complete dish, which simultaneously provides good protein (egg), energy complex carbohydrates (buckwheat), and vegetables. Thanks to spinach, it is particularly rich in beta-carotene (100% of the recommended daily intake of an adult), vitamins C and B9

(50% of the recommended intake). It also provides a quarter of the daily needs of fiber and calcium.
- Not very fat, it has a reasonable energy intake: 290 kcal, it is suitable for overweight.
- In cases of high cholesterol, remember to count the egg in your weekly quota.

CUPS OF STRAWBERRIES WITH MANGO

INGREDIENTS

- 400g strawberries
- 1 mango
- 60g frozen blackcurrant kernels
- 2 teaspoons honey all flowers
- 4 tablespoons of homemade pressed orange juice or fresh ray
- 1 tablespoon of silver-colored sugar pearls
- 4 lace pancakes

DIRECTIONS

1. A few hours in advance, place the black currants in the refrigerator to thaw.
2. Wash the strawberries under running water, pat them thoroughly with paper towels, and shake them off. Wash the mango under running water and sponge it.
3. Mix the honey with the orange juice.
4. Cut the mango in half (cut flush with the core). Peel each half and cut into cubes. Cut the strawberries in half. Delicately mix mango, strawberries, blackcurrant, and orange sauce. Divide the fruit salad into 4 cups. Garnish with sugar pearls, and arrange a lace crepe in each cup. Enjoy it immediately.

Nutritional interest

The strawberry mango cut combines 4 fruits richest in vitamin C so that a serving represents 80% of the recommended daily intake to an adult. It is also a healthy source of beta-carotene (especially thanks to mango), vitamin B9, and fiber: 15% of the recommended intake for each of these nutrients.

Providing potassium and simple sugars based on fruits with alkalizing virtues, it can be offered in recovery after an effort to children or adult athletes.

Coconut-pineapple mousse

INGREDIENTS

- 3 eggs
- 37.5 cl of coconut milk
- 60g of sugar
- 1/4 to 1/3 pineapple (200g net)
- 5 half-sheets of gelatin
- 1 pinch of salt

DIRECTIONS

1. Separate the yolks and egg whites.
2. Soak the gelatin in a bowl of cold water.
3. Whip the egg yolks with the sugar. Gradually add the coconut milk. Put everything into a saucepan and cook on low heat, constantly stir until the cream is tableclothed.
4. Drain the gelatin carefully, and add it to the coconut cream. Whip, and as soon as the gelatin is dissolved, remove the pan from the heat. Let cool for 1 hour in the refrigerator.
5. Peel the pineapple: remove its skin. It's the central hard part and its "eyes." Make sure you have 200g of flesh that you cut into small cubes.
6. Add a pinch of salt to the egg whites and beat in the snow firmly. Mix them gently with the coconut cream. Add the

pineapple dice. Divide the mousse into 4 ramekins and put in, at least, 2 hours in the refrigerator before eating.

Nutritional interest

Thanks to coconut milk—the coconut-pineapple mousse is rich in potassium, vegetable iron, and vitamin B5. Thanks to the eggs, it provides proteins of excellent nutritional quality. Coconut milk is good and high in saturated fat (17%), but it is mainly lauric acid, which, according to recent studies, does not affect the blood cholesterol level.

Spinach gratin with goat cheese

INGREDIENTS

- 250g fresh spinach
- 1 teaspoon of butter (10 g)
- 1 teaspoon flour (10 g)
- 10 cl of goat's milk
- 30g fresh goat cheese
- Nutmeg
- Salt pepper

DIRECTION

1. Wash the spinach under running water, sponge them out, mop them up. Place them in a pan with salt and pepper, cover, cook on low heat for 15 minutes.
2. Preheat the oven to 200° C.
3. Place the butter and sifted the flour in a saucepan. Mix over low heat. Add the milk gradually. Salt and pepper, grate some nutmeg. Cook over low heat, constantly stir for some minutes.
4. Mix the bechamel with the well-drained spinach. Arrange everything in an individual gratin dish, and emit the goat cheese over it — Bake in the oven for some minutes.

Nutritional interest

Thanks to spinach, this gratin is rich in vegetable iron, vitamins E and K, anti-oxidant carotenoids, and fiber. Enriched with milk and goat cheese, it provides nearly 400 mg of calcium or 45% of the recommended daily intake to an adult. This dish is particularly suitable for children, teenagers, pregnant women (if you choose a cheese made from pasteurized milk), and the elderly.

Eggs with milk and goat cheese

INGREDIENTS

- Two eggs
- 40 cl whole goat's milk
- 60g Pouligny-Saint-Pierre (goat cheese)
- Two slices of Bayonne ham (60g)
- Pepper

DIRECTIONS

1. Preheat the oven to 180° C.
2. Cut the cheese into small cubes. Slice the ham in chiffonade.
3. Beat the eggs in an omelet. Add the milk gradually. Add the diced goat cheese, ham, and a little pepper.
4. Divide the resulting preparation into four individual ramekins. Arrange the ramekins in an oven dish in which you have poured the bottom of the water so that the milk eggs cook in a bain-marie.
5. Bake for 30 minutes at 180 ° C. Check the cooking of the eggs with a knife tip (the preparation does not stick when the eggs are cooked).

Nutritional interest

Milk and goat eggs are rich in high-quality protein for growth, as well as muscle maintenance. Can be served as a main dish, or for replacing the meat.

Thanks to milk and goat cheese. They provide vitamins B2, B12, A, and D, as well as calcium: 150 mg per serving, or 17% of the recommended daily intake.

They are especially suitable for children, teens, athletes, and the elderly.

Palets with squash seeds

INGREDIENTS

- 80g flour type 55 or 80
- 5 tablespoons of olive oil
- 1/2 teaspoon of baking soda (yeast)
- 40g squash seeds
- 30g dried tomatoes
- 1 teaspoon dried oregano
- Salt

DIRECTIONS

1. Mix the flour, baking soda, squash seeds, sun-dried tomatoes, and oregano. Include 4 tablespoons of olive oil and 1 pinch of salt. Add a few spoons of water to form a ball of dough. Let stand, at least, 30 minutes at room temperature.
2. Preheat the oven to 180° C. Arrange a sheet of baking paper on a baking sheet. Brush with the remaining oil.
3. Sprinkle with flour the work plan. Roll out the dough as finely as possible with a rolling pin. Use a cookie cutter to cut pucks. Arrange the pucks on the parchment paper. Bake for 15 minutes at 185° C. Check the cooking with a knife tip (the dough does not stick when the puck is cooked).

Nutritional interest

- The squash seeds combine healthy ingredients, useful in cardiovascular prevention: olive oil and squash seeds, high in unsaturated fats that help reduce the level of bad blood cholesterol and tomatoes, including lycopene (which colors them in red) is a powerful antioxidant.
- In case of diabetes, know that a portion of these pucks corresponds to 30g of bread.

Whiting Bread With Sesame

INGREDIENT

- 400g whiting fillets
- 4 tablespoons sesame oil
- 1 lemon
- 1 tablespoon soy sauce
- 1 clove of garlic
- 2 tablespoons minced lemongrass
- 1 small piece of ginger 1 cm
- 4 tablespoons sesame seeds
- 2 eggs
- Salt pepper

DIRECTIONS

1. Wash the lemon under running water, sponge it, squeeze it. Peel and slice the clove of garlic. Pass the ginger under the water, sponge it, and then grate it.
2. Prepare a marinade with two tablespoons of sesame oil, lemon juice, soy sauce, lemongrass, garlic, ginger, and a little pepper. Arrange the whiting fillets in the marinade and reserve them in the refrigerator for 2 hours.

3. Then carefully drain the fish fillets. Cook them for 5 minutes, then steam.
4. Separate the egg whites from the yolks. Spread each fillet of whiting in the egg yolk, and then in the sesame seeds to form a breadcrumb. Salt slightly. Quickly pass the breaded fish fillets in a non-stick frying pan with the remaining 2 spoons of oil. As soon as the sesame seeds are golden brown, stop cooking. Enjoy it immediately.

Nutritional interest

Whiting is rich in protein of excellent quality for growth, as is the maintenance of muscle mass. Breaded with sesame, it is also an excellent source of calcium, magnesium, and iron. It is suitable for hypercholesterolemia since sesame provides mainly unsaturated fats.

Almond/Pear Express Cream

INGREDIENTS

- 1 pot of semi-skimmed milk cheese with 3% fat
- 1 teaspoon of almond powder
- 1/2 teaspoon of flax seeds
- 2 drops of bitter almond extract
- 1 teaspoon of honey
- 1 lemon
- 1 pear
- 1 small square of dark chocolate

DIRECTIONS

1. Place the flax seeds in a non-stick pan. Roast them for 2 minutes over medium heat, then stir so that they do not burn.
2. Wash the lemon under running water, sponge it, and squeeze it.

3. Mix the white cheese with almond powder, bitter almond extract, 2 teaspoons lemon juice, honey, and flax seeds.
4. Wash the pear, peel it, dice it, and lemon it. Mix with almond cream.
5. Slice the chocolate into thin chips and sprinkle the cream. Enjoy it immediately.

Nutritional interest

The almond/pear cream is a good source of calcium, particularly recommended for growing young people or seniors in the prevention of osteoporosis. Rich in fiber, and it is satisfying and useful to regularise the transit. Thanks to flaxseed, it provides 50% of the recommended daily intake of essential Omega 3. As almonds mainly contain monounsaturated fats (the same as in olive oil), it can be supported in cases of hypercholesterolemia.

Seasonal vegetable cake

INGREDIENTS

- 100 g of flour type 55
- 2 eggs
- 3 tablespoons of olive oil
- 300g of already cooked vegetables: carrots, cauliflower, zucchini, broccoli, spinach, peas.
- 80 ml of semi-skimmed milk
- 1/2 sachet of yeast
- 40g of goat cheese
- 40g of Emmentaler
- 1 teaspoon chopped parsley
- 1 teaspoon chopped mint
- Salt pepper

DIRECTIONS

1. Heat the oven to 200° C. Line a small cake tin with parchment paper.
2. Quickly pass the vegetables in the pan with 1 spoon of oil to lightly grill. Season them with the herbs.
3. Mix the flour with the yeast, then the eggs. Gradually add the milk and the remaining 2 spoons of oil. Add salt and pepper. Finish by incorporating vegetables, diced goat cheese, and grated Emmental cheese.
4. Pour the mix into the cake pan and bake for 30 minutes. Check the cooking with a knife tip (when the cake is cooked, the dough does not stick to the knife).

Nutritional interest

- The seasonal vegetable cake is an energy starter, rich in complex carbohydrates and protein.
- In case of diabetes, one serving replaces 40g of bread (1/6 of baguette) or 100g of starch (3 tablespoons). In the case of hypercholesterolemia, avoid consuming other cheese during the day.

Zucchini flan

INGREDIENTS

- 1 zucchini
- 1 tomato
- 1 shallot
- 1 teaspoon of olive oil
- 1 pinch of oregano
- 1 egg
- 2 tablespoons cottage cheese
- 1 tablespoon thick cream
- 1 teaspoon Maïzena
- 1 tablespoon grated Emmental cheese
- Salt pepper

DIRECTIONS

1. Wash the zucchini and tomato under running water, pat, and peel them. Remove the fibrous central part of the tomato and cut it into quarters. Cut the zucchini into thin slices.
2. Peel and chop the shallot. Sweat over reasonably low heat in olive oil for a few minutes, then add the zucchini and tomato. Add salt, pepper, and oregano, then cover and cook for 15 minutes on low heat. At the end of cooking, discover the vegetables to reduce them well.
3. Preheat the oven to 180° C. Beat the omelet egg and mix it with the Fromage blanc, the cream, and the Maïzena. Add salt and pepper.
4. Place the vegetables in the bottom of an individual gratin dish. Cover them with gratin and sprinkle with grated cheese — Bake for 15 minutes at 180° C.

Nutritional interest

The zucchini custard is a complete dish, and it's perfect with a slice of bread and fruit for a balanced meal.

It helps to provide good protein (egg, cottage cheese, Emmental) to those who have difficulty in eating meat, including the elderly.

Mushroom cake ao-nori

INGREDIENTS

- 80g of buckwheat flour
- 5 eggs
- 600g mushrooms from Paris
- 2 shallots
- 2 cloves garlic
- 2 tablespoons olive oil
- 40g of ao-nori (green algae) in the jar

- 1 tablespoon chopped parsley
- 1 tablespoon of sunflower oil
- Salt pepper

DIRECTIONS

1. Prepare the dough by mixing the buckwheat flour with 20 cl of water, a nice pinch of salt, and 1/4 egg beaten into an omelet. Cover the salad bowl and let the dough rest in the refrigerator for 1 hour.
2. Drain and slice the ao-nori. Peel and slice garlic and shallots. Wash the mushrooms under running water, remove their earthy foot, cut them into slices. In a pan, sauté garlic, shallots, and mushrooms with olive oil. Salt and pepper, sprinkle with ao-nori. Cook for 10 minutes (all the mushrooms water must be evaporated) and add the parsley.
3. Bake 4 patties in a lightly greased non-stick pan with an oiled brush.
4. Spread the pan-fried mushrooms on 4 patties. Iron each pancake in the pan. Break an egg in the center. Once the white is cooked, fold the edges of the cake to give it a square shape, and then serve it immediately.

Nutritional interest

- The mushroom cake ao-nori is a complete dish: it provides complex energy carbohydrates (flour), proteins (eggs), and fiber (mushrooms, algae). Thanks to the ao-nori. It is a good source of iron and iodine.
- Its energy intake is reasonable: 280 kcal per galette.
- It can be consumed in the case of the celiac disease since buckwheat does not contain gluten.

Vegetable toast

INGREDIENTS

- 30g chickpeas
- 1 big tomato "Heart of beef" (200 to 250g)
- 30g red pepper
- 1 clove of garlic
- 1 teaspoon chopped parsley
- 3 teaspoons of olive oil
- 1/2 teaspoon chopped basil
- 1 nice slice of country bread (50 to 60g)
- Salt pepper

DIRECTIONS

1. Soak the chickpeas in cold water for an hour. The next day, drain them carefully and allow them to dry thoroughly before cooking.
2. Peel the garlic. Wash the piece of pepper, remove its whitish fibrous parts and seeds. Wash the tomato, remove the fibrous central part.
3. Mix the chickpeas, the clove of garlic, the piece of pepper, 50 g of tomato, the parsley, salt, and pepper. Shape the slab-shaped dough the size of the minced steak and pan fry with 2 tablespoons olive oil 3 minutes on each side.
4. Grill the slice of country bread.
5. Cut the remaining tomato into carpaccio.
6. Arrange half of the tomato carpaccio on the slice of bread, drizzle with olive oil, season with salt, pepper, and basil. Put over the chickpea galette. Finish with the rest of the carpaccio season. Enjoy it immediately.

Nutritional interest

Vegetable bread is a complete balanced dish. It is rich in protein, energy complex carbohydrates (bread, chickpeas), fiber, vitamin C, and anti-oxidant lycopene (tomato). It combines many ingredients of the Mediterranean diet, protectors of the cardiovascular system.

Peach fondant

INGREDIENTS

- 2 pears Conference
- 2 eggs
- 1/4 liter of semi-skimmed milk
- 2 tablespoons maple syrup or 3 teaspoons of sugar
- 1 lemon
- 30g oat flakes
- 1 vanilla pod
- 2 tablespoons rum
- 2 level tablespoons of flaked almonds

DIRECTIONS

1. Spread the vanilla pod under the water, then slice it in half and place it with the milk in a saucepan. Heat to a boil, then turn off the heat and let the vanilla brew.
2. Preheat the oven to 180° C.
3. Mix the oatmeal. Remove the vanilla pod from cooled milk, and gradually mix milk and oatmeal. Add the maple syrup, the rum, then the two beaten egg omelet.
4. Wash the lemon and squeeze it. Wash the pears, cut them in half, remove the fibrous central part and the pips, peel them. Lemon them immediately to avoid blackening them. Arrange the four half-pears in a gratin dish. Pour over the milk mixture.
5. Bake for 30 minutes at 180° C. Check the cooking with a knife tip.
6. Quickly brown the flaked almonds in a non-stick frying pan and decorate the fondant.

Nutritional interest

Not very sweet, high in fiber with pears and oatmeal, this low-glycemic dessert is suitable for diabetes. Providing only 190 kcal per serving, it can also be consumed in case of overweight.

Exotic fruit verrines

INGREDIENTS

- 2 kiwis
- 1 mango
- 1/2 grenade
- 1/4 liter of semi-skimmed milk
- 2 eggs
- 25g of sugar
- 1 vanilla pod
- 2 half-sheets of gelatin or 1/2 teaspoon of agar agar

DIRECTIONS

1. Wash the vanilla pod, slice it in half, and place it in a saucepan with the milk. Heat and stop the fire just before boiling. Let the vanilla steep in the milk.
2. Position the gelatin in a bowl of cold water.
3. Separate the whites and egg yolks. Whip the yolks with the sugar. Add the cooled and filtered milk. Pour everything into the saucepan and cook on low heat, continually stirring until the cream thickens. Add drained half-leaves of gelatin or agar-agar, wait for their complete dissolution to cut the fire. Divide the custard into four glasses and refrigerate for at least 2 hours.
4. Wash the fruits under running water and sponge them out. Peel the kiwis and mango, and cut them into cubes. Collect the grains from the pomegranate. Mix these fruits gently and divide them into the glasses. Enjoy it immediately.

Shortbread with jam

INGREDIENTS

- 100g of wheat flour type 55
- 50g butter or margarine rich in omega 3 not lightened
- 50g of sugar
- 1 egg
- 120g of strawberry or apricot jam, homemade if possible
- 2 tablespoons icing sugar
- 1 large star-shaped cookie cutter
- 1 round-shaped cookie cutter 1.5 cm in diameter

DIRECTIONS

1. Separate the whites from the egg yolk.
2. In a bowl, mix the flour, sugar, and butter until you have a texture of sand. Add the egg yolk to mix the dough ball. Let the dough rest in the refrigerator for at least 30 minutes.
3. Preheat the oven to 180 ° C. Arrange a sheet of baking paper on a baking sheet.
4. Spread the dough. Cut star-shaped shortbread. In half of these shortbreads, cut a small circle of dough in the middle.
5. Arrange the shortbread on the plate and bake for 15 minutes.
6. Let the shortbread a little cool. Cover each shortbread with jam and sprinkle each shortbread with icing sugar. Arrange the shortbreads pierced over jammed biscuits.

Nutritional interest

- Made with flour and jam. These biscuits are rich in carbohydrates and energy. They have their place at the end of a meal without starch or snack after a light lunch. They can also be used as a snack, in recovery after a sports training.

- Low in fat, they are suitable for hypercholesterolemia.

Chocolate Pear Charlotte

INGREDIENTS

- 18 biscuits with a spoon
- 1 tablespoon liquid vanilla extract
- 2 beautiful ripe pears
- 2 jars of chocolate cream-dessert (250g)
- 1 lemon
- 1 tablespoon chocolate granules

DIRECTIONS

1. Wash the lemon under running water, sponge it, and squeeze it.
2. Wash the pears, peel them, and remove any excessively ripe parts. Cut them into cubes. Place them in a small saucepan with the lemon juice. Cook them covered over low heat for 20 minutes. At the end of cooking, crush them in the sauce.
3. Mix the vanilla extract with 4 tablespoons of water. Dip the biscuits very quickly in the vanilla and line the bottom and edges of 4 ramekins. Spread half of the cooled compote on the biscuits. Pour over the chocolate cream (a 1/2 pot per ramekin). Finish with the remaining compote. Place the charlottes in the refrigerator for at least 4 hours.
4. Unmould the charlottes before serving and decorate them with chocolate granules.

Nutritional interest

- The charlotte pear/chocolate is a dessert or energetic snack rich in carbohydrates. Thanks to the pears. It has edible fiber and potassium content.
- Very low fat, it is suitable for hypercholesterolemia.

- It provides 250 kcal per serving: if you watch your line, take it at the end of a meal without starch.

Poached apricots with blackcurrant

INGREDIENTS

- 2 apricots
- 10 cl of pure blackcurrant juice
- 1 slice of gingerbread
- 1/2 vanilla pod
- 2 teaspoons of aspartame or sucralose powder

DIRECTIONS

1. Rinse the vanilla bean under running water and cut in half.
2. Place the blackcurrant juice and vanilla in a small saucepan. Heat until the first tremors, then let the vanilla brew, at least, 30 minutes.
3. Wash the apricots, pit them, and separate the mumps. Place them in the blackcurrant juice and let them cook for 15 minutes over low heat.
4. At the end of cooking, add the sweetener, remove the vanilla, and then discover the pan so that the blackcurrant juice is reduced.
5. Arrange the slice of gingerbread on a dessert plate. Add the apricot mumps. Sprinkle with blackcurrant syrup.
6. Allow cooling well before eating.

Nutritional interest

- Based on apricots and cassis, this dessert is rich in anti-oxidants: beta-carotene (pro-vitamin A) and anthocyanins (dark red pigments) that act synergistically in the body. "Sweet" with a sweetener, it has a reasonable energy intake: 145 kcal per serving.

- For a balanced meal, precede your poached apricots with meat, fish, and vegetables (or mixed salad) and dairy.

Bavarian vanilla/coffee

INGREDIENTS

- 1/2 liter of semi-skimmed milk
- 4 egg yolks
- 3 tablespoons of aspartame-based sweetener or sucralose
- 1 vanilla pod
- 2 teaspoons instant coffee
- 4 half -sheets of gelatin
- 1 tablespoon flaked almonds

DIRECTIONS

1. Soak 2 half-sheets of gelatin in a bowl of cold water.
2. Heat 1/4 liter of milk with the vanilla pod. When boiling, remove the milk from the heat and let the vanilla brew while it cools.
3. Separate the whites and yolks from 2 eggs.
4. Whisk the yolks, place them in a saucepan and add the cooled milk gradually. Cook this mixture on low heat, constantly stir until the cream coats the spoon. Remove the vanilla bean and add half of the sweetener and the drained gelatin. Whip until the perfect dissolution of the gelatin.
5. Divide the vanilla cream into four ramekins and refrigerate for 2 hours.
6. Prepare another coffee cream which you will pour gently into the ramekins and retake 2 hours.
7. Just before serving, quickly pass the almonds in a nonstick skillet for browning and decorating the bavarois.

Nutritional interest

Bavarian is rich in calcium (milk) and protein (milk, egg). Based on semi-skimmed milk and sweetener, its calorie intake is reasonable: 115 kcal per serving. Without sugar, it is suitable for people with diabetes. In case of high cholesterol, consider counting the yolk among your eggs of the week.

Clafoutis multi fruits

INGREDIENTS

- 400g (net) of seasonal fruits: peaches, apricots, cherries
- 20 cl of semi-skimmed milk
- 2 eggs
- 40g flour (2 tablespoons)
- 40g sugar (2 tablespoons)
- 1 teaspoon liquid vanilla extract

DIRECTIONS

1. Wash the fruits under running water. Stake and pit the cherries. Peel the peaches. If the fruit is very ripe, remove any damaged parts. Cut them into small cubes.
2. Preheat the oven to 180° C.
3. Beat the omelet eggs and add the sugar. Then gradually add the sifted flour. Finish with milk and vanilla extract.
4. Mix the clafoutis with the fruits. Pour the mixture into an oven pan. Bake for 180° C for 30 minutes: check the cooking with a knife tip or a baking needle (the clafoutis is cooked when its dough does not stick to the tip of the knife).

Nutritional interest

- Clafoutis multi fruits can take advantage of the good fruit nutrients (except vitamin C degraded by heat): fiber, potassium, beta-carotene, and antioxidant polyphenols. Thanks to eggs and milk, it provides good quality protein and calcium. It is an interesting dessert for children or teenagers who have difficulty eating fruit at the table.

- Its energy intake is reasonable: 225 kcal the portion.

Leek gratin

INGREDIENTS

- 2 leeks
- 1 teaspoon of butter
- 1 teaspoon Maïzena
- 12 cl of whole milk
- 50g grated Emmental cheese
- Nutmeg
- Salt pepper

DIRECTIONS

1. Wash the leeks carefully; remove their earthy foot and their green. Cut the whites into pieces and place them in a steamer. Salt them and cook for 25 minutes. Once cooked, let them drain well.
2. Preheat the grill in the oven.
3. Mix the butter and Maïzena. Place them over low heat in a small saucepan to obtain a white roux. Add the milk with a whisk.
4. Add grated nutmeg and half of the Emmental cheese at the end of cooking. Salt lightly and pepper.
5. Arrange the leeks in the bottom of an individual gratin dish. Cover with Mornay sauce and sprinkle with remaining Emmental cheese.

Nutritional interest

- Thanks to milk and Emmental, leek gratin is very rich in calcium: (600 mg per serving, or 50% of the recommended intake for over 50s) and protein of excellent quality.

- Thanks to leeks, it also provides fiber, potassium, and carotenoids with antioxidant properties.
- This dish is particularly adapted to the needs of teenagers, pregnant women, and seniors.

Gluten-free chocolate fondant

INGREDIENTS

- 100g of dark chocolate pastry
- 50g of butter
- 50g of sugar
- 1 egg
- 40g of Maïzena
- 1 teaspoon of natural vanilla extract
- 4 individual non-stick molds

DIRECTIONS

1. Heat the oven to 180° C.
2. Separate the whites from the egg yolk. Add a pinch of salt to the whites and beat in the snow.
3. Cut the chocolate into squares and butter into cubes. Place these two ingredients in a large bowl and microwave in the oven for 1 minute to melt. Mix them thoroughly with a whisk.
4. Mix the egg yolk with the sugar. Add the sifted Maïzena, beat well. Then add the chocolate and butter mixture, as well as the vanilla extract. Finally, gently add the white to snow.
5. Divide the dough into the 4 molds — Bake for 10 minutes at 180° C.

Light tomato pie

INGREDIENTS

- 4 sheets of brick
- 600g tomatoes
- 1 beautiful onion
- 1 clove of garlic
- 3 tablespoons of olive oil
- 2 tablespoons of a dry white wine
- 1 bouquet garni
- 1 teaspoon of Provence herbs
- 4 eggs
- 1 mozzarella ball
- Salt pepper

DIRECTIONS

1. Peel and slice garlic and onion. Wash the tomatoes under running water, peel them, remove the fibrous core, and cut them into wedges.
2. Fry garlic, onion, and tomatoes in 2 tablespoons olive oil. Add the white wine, the bouquet garni, the herbs of Provence, salt, and pepper. Cover and simmer on low heat for 20 minutes. Add some water during cooking if necessary, and let reduce at the end of cooking. Take off the bouquet garni.
3. Preheat the thermostat oven 6/7 (200 ° C).
4. Position a sheet of parchment paper in the bottom of a pie plate for four people. Cover with a sheet of brick that you brush with olive oil with a brush. Arrange the other three sheets of brick in the same way.
5. Mix the tomato coulis with the beaten egg omelet. Correct the seasoning if necessary. Arrange this device on the filo paste. Finish with the sliced mozzarella. Bake 15 minutes.

Nutritional interest

The light tomato pie is a complete dish, providing proteins (eggs, mozzarella), complex carbohydrates (brick sheets), fibers and anti-oxidants (tomatoes) simultaneously. Its calorie intake is reasonable: 295 kcal per serving, it is suitable for overweight.

Omelet with Cottage Cheese and Fruits

INGREDIENT

- 2 eggs
- 1 tbsp. (15 mL) water
- 1/4 cup (60 mL) low-sodium cottage cheese
- 1/2 cup (125 mL) drained canned fruit mingue
- icing sugar (optional)

DIRECTIONS

1. Whisk eggs and water in a bowl.
2. Spray an 8-inch (20 cm) nonstick skillet with cooking spray. Heat the pan over medium heat. Pour in the egg mixture. As the eggs begin to cook near the wall, using a spatula, gently scrape the cooked portions towards the center. Bend and turn the pan to allow the uncooked egg to flow into the free space.
3. When eggs are cooked on top but still wet, evenly spread the cottage cheese in the center of the omelet. Using a spoon, place a cup of fruit Macedonia on the cheese. Fold each side of the omelet towards the center and the fruit Macedonia.
4. Slide the omelet on a plate. Sprinkle with 1/4 cup of the fruit Macedonia and, if desired, sift icing sugar.

French toast with apples and mint

INGREDIENTS

- 2 eggs, beaten lightly
- 1/8 tsp. at t. (1/2 mL) mint

- ½ cup (125 mL) milk
- ¾ cup (175 mL) applesauce
- 4 slices white bread

PREPARATION

1. In a bowl, combine eggs, milk, and mint.
2. Add the applesauce to the mixture.
3. Melt some margarine in a nonstick skillet over medium-high heat.
4. Dip the bread slices in the mixture and place it in the pan.
5. When the side of the bread facing down is brown, return the slice, and cook the other side.
6. Garnish with syrup.

Apple and Mint French Toast, 5.0 out of 5 based on 1 rating

Breakfast Burrito

INGREDIENTS

- Non-stick cooking spray
- 4 eggs
- 3 tablespoons chopped green peppers
- ¼ tsp. ground cumin
- ½ teaspoon chili sauce
- 2 flour tortillas, burrito size
- 2 tablespoons salsa

PREPARATION

1. In a bowl, beat the eggs, green peppers, cumin, and chili sauce.
2. Pour in the pan and cook, stirring for one to two minutes until the eggs are cooked.

3. Heat the tortillas for 20 seconds in the microwave or another pan over medium heat.
4. Place half of the egg filling on each tortilla and roll like a burrito.
5. Serve each burrito with a tablespoon of salsa.

Spinach and ricotta cheese frittata

INGREDIENTS

- 10 eggs Omega-3
- 1 cup ricotta cheese
- 1 tbsp. to s. fresh herbs, chopped
- 1 tbsp. to s. olive oil
- 1 medium onion, chopped
- 1 clove garlic, finely chopped
- 2 cups raw spinach

PREPARATION

1. Heat oven to 350 ° F.
2. Sauté onion and garlic in olive oil in a non-stick ovenproof pan.
3. -Add the spinach and sauté until they wither.
4. -Mix eggs, ricotta cheese, and fresh herbs.
5. -Add the egg mixture to the pan.
6. -Finish the cooking of the frittata in the oven (about 10 minutes or until the top is completely seized).
7. -Serve hot.

Omelette and summer vegetables

INGREDIENTS

- Nonstick cooking spray

- 1/4 cup frozen whole grain corn, thawed
- 1/3 cup chopped zucchini
- 3 tablespoons chopped green onion
- 2 tablespoons water
- 1/4 tsp black pepper or 1 tablespoon / 4 teaspoonful of Mrs. Extra Spicy Dash
- 2 Large Egg Whites
- 1 Large Whole Egg
- 1 ounce Low Fat Cheddar Cheese

PREPARATION

1. Heat a small saucepan over medium-high heat. Coat the pan with the cooking spray. Add the corn, zucchini, and onions to the pan; sauté 4 minutes, or until vegetables are tender and still firm. Remove from fire. Heat a 10-inch frying pan over medium-high heat.
2. Combine water, pepper (or Mrs. Dash), egg whites and egg in a bowl, and mix well with a whisk. Coat the pan with cooking spray. Pour the egg mixture into the pan; cook until edges are set (about 2 minutes).
3. Gently lift the edges of the omelet with a spatula, tilt the pan so that the uncooked egg mixture comes into contact with the pan. Using a spoon, place the vegetable mixture on one half of the omelet, and then sprinkle the cheese mixture with vegetables.
4. Take off the omelet with the spatula and fold the omelet on itself (in half). Bake two more minutes or until cheese has melted. Slowly slide the omelet onto a plate.

Blueberry pancakes

INGREDIENTS

- 1 1/2 cups sifted all-purpose flour
- 2 tbsp. yeast tea
- 3 tbsp. sugar soup
- 1 cup buttermilk
- 2 tbsp. melted salt-free margarine soup
- 2 lightly beaten eggs
- 1 cup rinsed or frozen, canned blueberries

PREPARATION

1. Sift the flour, yeast, and sugar together in a large mixing bowl.
2. Dig a hole in the middle of the flour mixture and add the other ingredients.
3. Start mixing from the center and gradually incorporate the flour until smooth. Start cooking immediately!
4. Heat a 12-inch frying pan and brush with oil.
5. Measure 1/3 cup pancake mixture; pour into pan and cook just once, turning pancake only once.

Roast pork with pineapple

INGREDIENTS

- 1 roast pork (about 3 lb. - 1.4 kg)
- Pepper
- 1/2 tsp. at t. crushed red peppers (if you like spicy food)
- 1 can of pineapple puree (8 oz)
- 2 Tbsp. to s. sugar or Splenda
- 1/2 tsp. to s. soy sauce with low sodium content
- 1 minced garlic clove
- 1/4 tsp. at t. dried basil
- 1 tbsp. to s. cornstarch
- 1/4 cup cold water
- 1 green pepper or diced red pepper

PREPARATION

1. Cut the roast in half if mandatory and place it in a slow cooker. Add pepper to taste.
2. Mix all the ingredients except cornstarch, water, and pepper; pour over the roast. Cover and cook for 8 to 10 hours at low temperature or 4 to 6 hours at high temperature.
3. Remove the roast and check the temperature with a meat thermometer.
4. Drain the pineapple and reserve the cooking sauce. Put the roast and pineapples back in the slow cooker.
5. Add water to the cooking sauce to make 3/4 cup. Pour into a pan.
6. Mix the cornstarch in the heated cooking sauce.
7. Add the pepper cut into cubes.
8. Cook, stirring until the mixture thickens. Pour over the roast; serve with rice according to your taste.

Roasted Spaghetti Squash with Kale and Parmesan

INGREDIENTS

- 1 large spaghetti squash
- 2 tbsp. 1 tbsp. extra virgin olive oil
- 2 tbsp. dried oregano
- 2 cloves minced garlic
- ½ tsp. dried chili flakes
- 1 large kale bunch (kale)
- ½ cup finely grated Parmesan cheese

PREPARATION

1. Preheat oven to 350ºF (180ºC).

2. Cut the spaghetti squash in half lengthwise. With a large spoon, scrape and remove the seeds that you could throw in the compost.

3. Place the two squash halves (cut side up) on a large baking tray and drizzle with 2 tbsp — a tablespoon of olive oil sprinkles with oregano, garlic, and flakes of chili peppers. Turn them on their cut side so that they can cook faster. Bake in the center of the oven until the squash is tender (prick with a fork) - approx. 45 minutes. Reserve and leave to cool for about 5 minutes. With a large spoon and fork, remove the flesh from the squash halves, and put in a large bowl. Work it gently to separate the strands so that it looks like spaghetti roughly.

4. On the other hand, you will have washed the kale from which you have removed the ribs and stems. Tear the leaves into pieces (about the size of a bite). Spin in the juicer, and then transfer the kale to a large bowl. Add the c. Olive oil and stir to lightly coat the pieces spread on two baking trays and roast until crisp and bright green - 12 to 14 minutes. Book.

5. To serve, place squash spaghetti on a large dish, and garnish with kale chips. Sprinkle with parmesan, salt, and pepper to taste.

Salad of grated carrots with lemon-dijon vinaigrette

INGREDIENTS

- 9 small carrots (14 cm), peeled
- 2 tbsp. Dijon mustard
- 1 tbsp. lemon juice
- 2 tbsp. extra virgin olive oil
- 1-2 tbsp. honey (to taste)
- ¼ tsp. Salt

- ¼ tsp. ground pepper (to taste)
- 2 Tbsp. chopped parsley
- One green onion, finely sliced

PREPARATION

1. Grate the carrots with the robot. Book.
2. In a bowl, mix Dijon mustard, lemon juice, honey, olive oil, salt, and pepper. Add carrots, fresh parsley, and green onions. Twist to coat well. Cover and refrigerate until ready to serve.

NOTE: if your carrots are more or less sweet, adjust the touch of honey.

Oriental Eggplant Dip with Grilled Pepper Steak

INGREDIENTS

Marinade for steak

- 1 tbsp. brown sugar
- 2 garlic cloves, minced
- 1 tbsp. crushed black peppercorns
- 1 tbsp. olive oil
- 2 lb sirloin steak

Oriental Eggplant Dip

- 1 large eggplant
- 2 tbsp. brown sugar
- 1 tbsp. rice vinegar
- 1 tbsp. tablespoons water
- 1 tbsp. vegetable oil
- 4 garlic cloves, finely chopped
- 1 tbsp. fresh ginger, finely chopped
- 4 green onions, chopped
- 1 tbsp. pepper paste

- 1 tbsp. sesame oil
- 2 tbsp. fresh coriander, chopped

PREPARATION

Marinade for steak

- In a bowl, combine the ingredients for the marinade. Dry the steak with a paper towel, brush with oil, and rub with the mixture. Marinate for at least an hour. Grill to the desired degree of cooking.

Eggplant Oriental Dip

- Grill aubergine in an oven preheated to 425 ° F for about 45 minutes. Peel the eggplant and chop it finely. In a small bowl, combine sugar, vinegar, and water. In a big skillet, sauté garlic, ginger, green onions, and chili paste until fragrant. Add the vinegar mixture. Bring to a boil and add the eggplant. To mix everything. Remove from heat and add sesame oil. Serve cold or at room temperature with a grilled steak.

Simmered Canadian style

INGREDIENTS

- 1 slice of 500 g (1.1 lb) of boneless and defatted beef paddle
- 2 tbsp. (30 ml) olive oil
- 1 cup onion, quartered
- 6 cloves of garlic, peeled
- 15 ml (1 tbsp) old-fashioned mustard
- 2 cup turnips, peeled and chopped quarters
- 1 cup carrots, cut in half lengthwise
- 4 cups green cabbage, quartered
- 1 liter (4 cups) chicken or beef broth

PREPARATION

1. In a skillet, brown the meat on each side in the oil. Place in the slow cooker. Book.
2. In the same pan, brown the onion quarters and garlic. Deglaze with a cup of broth and add mustard. Pour into the slow cooker, and add the rest of the ingredients.
3. Cover and cook at Low (Low) for about 8 hours or until meat is flaked with a fork. Adjust the seasoning to your taste.

Eggplant curry and chickpeas

INGREDIENTS

- 2 small eggplants
- 2 tbsp. tablespoon of sunflower oil
- 1 tbsp. brown or black mustard seeds
- 10-12 curry leaves
- 2 finely chopped onions
- 2 chopped dried peppers (to taste!)
- 4 Tbsp. garam masala
- 2 tsp. ground coriander
- 2 tbsp. turmeric
- 200 ml reduced-salt vegetable broth
- 200 ml yogurt, plain, low-fat
- 3 quartered tomatoes
- 400g canned chickpeas, rinsed and drained

PREPARATION

1. Cut the aubergines in half and then half in length. Heat 1/2 tsp. oil in large skillet and brown half of eggplant pieces for 2-3 minutes, turning until browned and crisp. Pour into a dish. Put some oil in the pan and repeat with remaining pieces of eggplant. Book.

2. Pour the remaining oil into the pan; add the mustard seeds and the curry leaves — Brown for 30 seconds until you smell the aromas. Add the onion; continue cooking until it begins to brown. Add the dried pepper and spices, then half of the yogurt. Cook 1 min longer, then add remaining yogurt, tomato wedges, and vegetable broth. Simmer over very low heat for 25 to 30 minutes until thickened.
3. Stir in chickpeas and eggplant. Simmer another 5 minutes or so for the mixture to be warm and eggplants well cooked and tender. Serve to your liking with rice or naan bread baked in the oven or seared with a little oil, sprinkled with a few finely chopped curry leaves.

Eggplant and chickpea bites

INGREDIENTS

- 3 large aubergines cut in half (make a few cuts in the flesh with a knife) Spray
- oil
- 2 large cloves garlic, peeled and deglazed
- 2 tbsp. coriander powder
- 2 tbsp. cumin seeds
- 400g canned chickpeas, rinsed and drained
- 2 Tbsp. chickpea flour
- Zest and juice of 1/2 lemon
- 1/2 lemon quartered for serving
- 3 tbsp. tablespoon of polenta

PREPARATION

1. Preheat the oven to 200ºC. Spray the eggplant halves generously with oil and place them on the meat side up on a baking sheet. Sprinkle with coriander and cumin seeds, and then place the cloves of garlic on the plate. Season and roast

for 40 minutes until the flesh of eggplant is completely tender. Reserve and let cool a little.

2. Scrape the flesh of the eggplant in a bowl with a spatula and throw the skins in the compost. Thoroughly scrape and make sure to incorporate spices and crushed roasted garlic. Add chickpeas, chickpea flour, zest, and lemon juice. Crush roughly and mix well, then check to season. Do not worry if the mixture seems a bit soft - it will firm up in the fridge.

3. Form about twenty pellets and place them on a baking sheet covered with parchment paper.

4. Preheat oven to 180ºC (rotating heat 160ºC. Remove the meatballs from the fridge and coat them by rolling them in the polenta. Place them back on the baking pan and spray a little oil on each. Roast for 20 minutes until golden and crisp. Serve with lemon wedges. You can also serve these dumplings with a spicy yogurt dip with harissa, this delicious but spicy mashed paste of hot peppers and spices from the Maghreb.

Iranian ash-e-jo soup with barley

INGREDIENTS

- 2 L chicken broth
- 2 tbsp. vegetable oil
- 1 medium onion, chopped
- 1 cup pearl barley
- 1 tbsp. turmeric
- 2 limes (1 pressed, 1 sliced into 8 wedges)
- 1/4 cup of salt-free tomato paste
- 1 cup carrots in small dice
- 1/2 cup sour cream
- 1/2 cup chopped fresh parsley

Preparation

1. Heat the chicken broth in a saucepan and let simmer.
2. In a large cauldron, fry onion until transparent in vegetable oil over medium heat. Add the pearl barley, stir for one minute, then stir in the hot chicken broth, turmeric, lime juice, tomato paste, salt, and pepper. Bring to a boil, reduce fire, and simmer for one hour.
3. Add the carrots and simmer over low heat for another 30 minutes or until the soup has thickened, and the carrots and barley are tender. If the soup is too thick, add a little hot water in small amounts.
4. Pour the sour cream into a bowl. Slowly add 1/2 cup of hot soup while whisking constantly. Gradually pour the mixture of sour cream and soup into the large cauldron mixing well.
5. Serve in bowls, sprinkle with chopped parsley and serve with limes.

Cranberry sauce with orange and ginger

INGREDIENTS
- 1 can of whole cranberry sauce
- ¼ cup of water
- 1 tablespoon of orange peel
- 1 teaspoon of grated ginger

PREPARATION:
1. Pour the sauce into a saucepan with the water, zest, and ginger
2. Bring to a low boil and stir over low heat for 3 minutes
3. Serve immediately on meat, or let cool and store in the fridge

Raspberry and peach smoothie

INGREDIENTS

- 1 cup frozen raspberries
- 1 peach, pitted and diced
- 1/2 cup tofu silky (or more, if needed)
- 1 tbsp. maple syrup or honey (or stevia or Splenda)
- 1 cup almond beverage, non-fortified

Preparation

1. Mix all the ingredients until you have a homogeneous texture.

Steamed Jamaican Fish

INGREDIENTS

- 4 tilapia fillets (100 g each fillet)
- 1/2 cup olive oil
- 3/4 cup red and green peppers, sliced
- 1/2 cup onion, chopped
- 1 / 4 c. black pepper téa
- 1 tbsp. téa with chili sauce
- 1 sprig of thyme
- 1 tbsp. Ketchup
- Juice 1/2 lime (1 tablespoon lime juice)
- 1 cup hot water

PREPARATION

1. Heat the oil in a skillet over medium heat and sauté the onion and peppers.
2. Add pepper, hot pepper sauce, thyme, ketchup, lime juice, and ½ cup warm water. Mix well.
3. Put the fish in the pan and add ½ cup of hot water. Cover the fish with sauce and vegetables with a spoon.

4. Cover the pan and cook for 5 minutes. Turn the fish over, cover, and cook for another 5 minutes, or until the fish is cooked.
5. Steamed Jamaican Fish, 3.0 out of 5 based on two ratings

Grilled turkey with lime

INGREDIENTS

- ½ cup (125 mL) Lime juice
- ¼ cup (60 mL) Vegetable oil
- 2 tbsp. (30 mL) Liquid Honey
- 1 Tbsp. (5 mL) Dried thyme leaves
- 1 tbsp. (5 mL) Dried rosemary
- 2/3 pound (300g) Turkey breast, skinless, and boneless

PREPARATION

1. Prepare the marinade by mixing the first five ingredients.
2. Reserve 2 tbsp. (30mL) marinade for basting.
3. Cut the breast in two slices over the thickness to make cutlets.
4. Add the escalopes to the marinade. Cover and refrigerate 1 - 2 hours.
5. Preheat oven grill at high power (500 ° F) or preheat grill.
6. Remove the brisket from the marinade.
7. In the oven or on the barbecue, grill the cutlets for 4 minutes on each side, or until they are cooked through.
8. Use the reserved marinade to brush the cutlets during cooking.
9. Discard the rest of the marinade.

Lemon juice can be used instead of lime juice.

This recipe can be made with two chicken breasts, skinless and boned (300g total) in place of the turkey.

Shrimp salad, sweet peas, and wasabi-lime vinaigrette

INGREDIENTS

- 1 pound large shrimp, shelled
- 2 cups sweet peas, trimmed
- 1 cup water chestnuts, drained
- 1 cup soy sprouts

Wasabi-Lime dressing

- 1/2 cup vegetable oil
- 1/4 cup rice vinegar
- 1 vs. to s. lime juice
- 3 tbsp.
- 1 teaspoon wasabi powder at t. sugar
- 1/2 tsp. at t. ginger, finely chopped
- 1/2 tsp. at t. garlic, finely chopped

PREPARATION

1. Put a large pot filled with water to a boil.
2. Add the shrimp and sweet peas, and cook until the shrimps turn pink (about 2 minutes).
3. Immediately transfer shrimp and sweet peas to ice water to stop cooking, then drain.
4. Combine vinaigrette by whipping all ingredients listed.
5. Mix shrimp, sweet peas, water chestnuts, and bean sprouts in vinaigrette and serve.

   Note: the wasabi powder is very spicy, moderate the amount for interesting spice!!!

Prawn salad, sweet peas and wasabi-lime vinaigrette, 1.5 out of 5 based on two ratings

Oatmeal and berry muffins

INGREDIENTS

- 1 cup (250 mL) non-blanched all-purpose flour
- ½ cup (125 mL) quick-cooking oatmeal 1/2 cup
- (160 mL) stuffed brown sugar
- 1/2 tbsp (1/2 cup) tea) baking soda
- 2 eggs
- 125 ml (1/2 cup) applesauce
- 60 ml (1/4 cup)
- orange canola oil 1, grated rind only
- 1 lemon, grated rind
- 15 ml (1 tbsp) lemon juice
- 180 ml (3/4 cup) fresh raspberries
- 180 ml (3/4 cup) fresh blueberries.

PREPARATION

1. Put the grill at the center of the oven. Preheat oven to 180° C (350° F). Line 12 muffin cups with paper or silicone trays.
2. In a bowl, combine flour, oatmeal, brown sugar, and baking soda. Book.
3. In a big bowl, whisk together eggs, applesauce, oil, citrus zest, and lemon juice. Add the dry ingredients to the wooden spoon. Add the berries and mix gently.
4. Spread the mixture in the boxes. Sprinkle top with pistachio muffins. Bake for 20 to 22 minutes or until a toothpick inserted in the center of a muffin comes out clean. Let cool.

Sautéed shrimp and apple

INGREDIENTS

- ½ lb (227 g) headless shrimp with shell
- ¾ apple (diced)
- 2 celery stalks (diced)
- ½ red pepper (small, diced)

- 2 tbsp. (30 mL)

Marinade vegetable oil

- 1/2 tsp. (2.5 mL) low sodium soy sauce
- 1 tbsp. tsp (5 mL) cornstarch
- Pinch of white pepper

Sauce

- 1/2 tsp. (2.5 mL) low sodium soy sauce
- 1 tbsp. teaspoon (5 mL) sugar
- 1 tbsp. (5 mL) cornstarch
- 2 tbsp. at the table (30 mL) cold water

PREPARATION

1. Remove shrimp shell and devein. Marinate the shrimp in the above marinade ingredients for 30 minutes.
2. Mix the ingredients of the sauce in a small bowl, mix well, and set aside.
3. Heat about 1 tablespoon of oil in a non-stick wok and sauté the shrimp until they turn pink. Remove them from the wok.
4. Heat about 1 tbsp. Oil in a non-stick wok sauté the celery briefly, then add the diced apple and red pepper, stirring until just cooked. Add shrimp and sauce and mix continuously until sauce thickens. Then serve.

Ma Po Tofu (Soy Cheese)

INGREDIENTS

- Ground lean pork (100 g or 3.5 oz)
- 1 block (350g) tofu (moderately firm, chopped ½ inch cubes)
- 2 cloves garlic (finely chopped)
- 1/4 fresh chili * (seeds removed, finely chopped)
- 1 tbsp. (15 mL) green onion (chopped)
- 1 tbsp. (15 mL) vegetable oil

Marinade

- 1 tsp. (15 mL) vegetable oil
- 1/2 tsp. (2.5 mL) low sodium soy sauce
- 1 tbsp. (5 mL) Chinese cooking wine
- 1 tbsp. (5 mL) sesame oil
- ½ tsp. 2 mL Sugar

Sauce

- 1/2 c. (2.5 mL) low sodium soy sauce
- 1 tbsp. (5 mL) sesame oil
- 3 Tbsp. tablespoons (45 mL) water
- 1 c. tablespoon (15 mL) cornstarch

PREPARATION

1. Mix the ingredients of the marinade. Add the minced pork and marinate for about 15 minutes.
2. Mix the sauce ingredients and set aside.
3. Heat the vegetable oil in a wok or skillet and fry the garlic and red pepper. Add the pork and sauté until the meat has completely cooked. Add the tofu and sauté over low heat until the ingredients are hot. Using a whisk, mix the sauce, constantly stir until the sauce thickens, then garnish with green onions and serve.

Rice pilaf with parsley

INGREDIENTS

- 1 cup (250 mL) white long-grain rice, uncooked
- 2 tbsp. (30 mL), Non-Hydrogenated Margarine
- 1 Medium, Onion, Chopped
- 1 ¾ cup (425 mL), Chicken Broth without Added Salt
- 2 Tbsp. (30 mL) Fresh chopped parsley

PREPARATION

1. Melt the margarine in a saucepan over medium heat. Add the chopped onion and sauté until softened. Add the rice and fry often until golden brown.
2. Add chicken broth and bring to a boil. Lower the heat and cover. Simmer the rice until tender and light.
3. Add parsley, mix, and then serve.
4. White rice can be substituted with basmati rice or parboiled rice. It will take longer cooking time for parboiled rice.

Thai beef salad

INGREDIENTS

- 1 C. (15 ml) cornstarch
- 1 tbsp. (15 mL) EACH grated fresh ginger and fresh lime juice
- Two cloves minced garlic
- 1 Tbsp. (5 mL) EACH sesame oil and Asian chili sauce
- 1 pound (454 g) sirloin steak, top sirloin steak or sliced loin
- 8 cup (s) (2 l) romaine lettuce shredded
- 4 tbsp. (20 mL) canola oil
- 1/2 cup (125 mL) half-grape tomatoes
- ½ cup (s) (125 mL) EACH cucumber julienne, yellow pepper strips, and red onion

Chilean vinaigrette with lime

- 1 c. (5 mL) grated lime zest
- 1/4 cup fresh lime juice
- 2 Tbsp. rice vinegar
- 1 C. (15 mL) EACH low-sodium soy sauce and liquid honey
- a stream of Asian chili sauce

PREPARATION

1. Combine in a large bowl, cornstarch, ginger, lime juice, garlic, sesame oil, and chili sauce. Add the beef and coat it thoroughly; let stand 10 minutes. Discard the marinade.
2. Meanwhile, heat 1 tbsp. (5 mL) Canola oil in big skillet or wok over medium-high heat. Sauté the tomatoes, cucumber, pepper, and onion until they have fallen, and then place them in a bowl. Heat the remaining oil and sauté the beef until browned and cooked. Add to vegetables and mix.
3. Whisk all the chili and lime vinaigrette ingredients together.
4. Add the vinaigrette to the skillet. Let it cook, stirring over medium heat until it is hot and slightly sticky while deglazing. Add enough salad vinaigrette to moisten, garnish with beef and reserved vegetables; drizzle with remaining vinaigrette.

Linguines with spicy shrimps

INGREDIENTS

- -12 shrimp of 31/40 caliber (it is also possible to use 6oz chicken breast cut into small pieces)
- -1 tbsp. canola oil
- -1 small minced garlic clove
- -1 pepperoncino or marinated jalapeño pepper
- -¼ cup prepared salsa (sweet, medium or spicy, to your
- liking) -¼ cup of cream of the table at 10 %
- -2 cups of linguine (or other dough of your choice) cooked
- -¼ cup chopped coriander

PREPARATION

1. Cook pasta as directed on the package.
2. While the pasta is cooking, sauté the shrimp in the oil in a medium-sized pan over medium-high heat.
3. When the shrimp begin to shoot the orange rose, add the garlic, pepperoncini, and prepared salsa.

4. Continue cooking over low heat until shrimp is cooked through.
5. When the pasta is ready, turn off the heat and add the cream and pasta to the shrimp mixture. Mix well to coat sauce pasta.
6. Garnish with fresh coriander and serve.

Kebabs of pork and pears grilled with honey

INGREDIENTS

- 1 lb (454g) Canadian pork (chop, shoulder or loin) boneless and well-defatted
- 1/2 cup (125 mL) apple juice
- 2 tbsp. 1 tbsp (30 mL) Dijon mustard
- 2 tbsp. honey
- 1 medium pear cut into wedges
- 1 medium red onion cut into 8 points
- 1 red or green pepper cut into 1 "/ 2.5 cm pieces
- 1 small sliced zucchini

PREPARATION

1. If the skewers used are bamboo, let them soak in water for one hour before cooking. Place pork cubes in a plastic bag that can be sealed in a bowl, but not made of metal or in a lidded container. In another bowl, mix apple juice, Dijon mustard, and honey. Pour this mixture over the pork cubes.
2. Remove the pork from the marinade. Pour the marinade into a small pan. Bring to a boil and let the marinade boil for at least a minute. Garnish the skewers alternating cubes of pork and pieces of pear, red onion, pepper, and zucchini.
3. Preheat the barbecue to the maximum temperature. Lightly oil barbecue surface before placing kebabs. Brush the kebabs with marinade. Close the barbecue and let the kebabs roast

over medium heat for 10 to 12 minutes, turning occasionally and continuing with the marinade. Accompany with rice.

Fresh berry salad with yogurt cream

INGREDIENTS

Berry salad:

- 250 ml (1 cup) red cherries, pitted and cut in half
- 250 ml (1 cup) blackberries
- 250 ml (1 cup) raspberries
- 250 ml (1 cup) blueberries
- 30 ml (2 tbsp. (30 mL) honey

Yogurt Cream:

- 500 mL (2 cups) plain Greek yogurt
- 60 mL (¼ cup) honey
- 15 mL (1 tablespoon) lemon juice

PREPARATION

1. In a bowl, mix the fruits with the honey. In a separate bowl, combine all the ingredients of the yogurt cream.
2. Spread yogurt in the center of each plate. Spread the fruit salad.
3. Fresh berry salad with yogurt cream, 4.5 out of 5 based on 2 ratings

Baba Ghanouj

INGREDIENTS

- 1 large aubergine, cut in half lengthwise
- 1 head of garlic, unpeeled
- 30 ml (2 tablespoons) of olive oil

- Lemon juice to taste

PREPARATION

1. Put the grill at the center of the oven. Preheat the oven to 350° F. Line a baking sheet with parchment paper.
2. Place the eggplant on the plate, skin side up. Roast until the meat becomes very tender and detaches easily from the skin. You can do this for about 1 hour, depending on the size of the eggplant. Let cool.
3. Meanwhile, cut the tip of the garlic cloves. Place the garlic cloves in a square of aluminum foil. Fold the edges of the sheet and fold together to form a tightly wrapped foil. Roast with the eggplant until tender, about 20 minutes. Let cool. Purée the pods with a garlic press.
4. With a spoon, scoop out the flesh of the eggplant and position it in the bowl of a food processor. Add the garlic puree, the oil, and the lemon juice. Stir until purée is smooth and pepper.
5. Serve with mini pita bread.

Curry turkey casserole

INGREDIENTS

- ¼ cup and 2 tbsp. canola oil or olive oil
- 1 small yellow onion, diced
- 2 cloves minced garlic
- ¼ cup all-purpose flour
- 1 cup 2% milk
- 2 cups chicken broth without added salt
- 2 tbsp. curry powder
- pepper
- 3 cups broccoli heads
- 1 cup chopped red peppers

- 4 cups cooked turkey cut into morceau inch pieces
- 3 cups medium sized cubed bread

PREPARATION

1. Preheat oven to 400 ° F. In a medium-sized cauldron, heat half cup canola oil over average heat. Put onion and garlic. Cook until softened before they turn golden about 7 minutes. Whisk, add the flour and continue to whisk for one minute. Slowly add the milk and chicken broth, stir continually until the mixture is creamy. Cook, frequently stir until you have a simmer sauce. Add the curry powder and season with pepper to taste. Add the broccoli heads and cook until the broccoli is starting to soften about 5 minutes. Add the turkey. Pour the mixture into an 8-inch square baking dish.
2. In a small bowl, pour 2 tbsp. Canola or olive oil on the cubes of bread, and mix well to coat evenly. Transfer the cubes of bread to the turkey mixture and cook in the oven until the sauce is bubbling and the bread becomes golden about 15 minutes.

Pasta with Mediterranean chicken in the pan

INGREDIENTS

- 2 zucchini, medium, raw, sliced
- 2 fresh tomatoes, diced
- 1 sweet red pepper, medium, diced
- 3 cloves garlic, minced
- 2 medium boneless chicken breasts, skinless (1 lb - 450 grams), cut into small pieces
- 1 tbsp. (15 ml) olive oil
- 1 tbsp. (5 mL) basil, dried
- 1/2 tsp. (2.5 ml) oregano leaf, dried

- 1/4 tsp. (1.25 ml) Rosemary, dried
- 1/2 tsp. (2.5 mL) freshly ground black pepper
- 2 1/2 cups (625 mL), chicken broth, low sodium
- 1/2 cup (125 mL) red or white wine (or use chicken broth)
- 2 cups (500 mL) dry pasta
- 2 tbsp. (10 mL) cornstarch
- 4 tbsp. (60 mL) parmesan cheese, grated
- 2 Tbsp. (30 mL) fresh parsley, chopped (optional garnish)

PREPARATION

1. Cut the zucchini into slices lengthwise and cut into semicircles. Cut tomatoes and red pepper into large cubes. Finely chop the garlic. Book everything.
2. Cut the chicken breasts into small pieces (about 1 to 2.5 cm each). Book.
3. Pour the olive oil in a large saucepan, put on high heat and reheat for one or two minutes. Stir in chicken and sauté for about 10 minutes until lightly browned. Stir occasionally.
4. Put the prepared zucchini, tomatoes, and red peppers in the same pan. Sprinkle with basil, oregano, rosemary, and black pepper. Stir and sauté for five to seven minutes over medium heat until vegetables are tender but still crisp. Leave the vegetables in the pan, but remove from heat.
5. Meanwhile, bring chicken broth and white wine to a boil in a saucepan over medium-high heat. Stir in the pasta and use a spoon to push the pasta to the bottom so that it is immersed in the broth. Thus ensure even cooking. Reduce to medium heat, and cook according to package directions, and until pasta is al dente as it will be heated again to the next step. Stir during cooking to prevent pasta from sticking.
6. Remove one cup (250 mL) broth from the pasta pan in a medium bowl and set aside. Stir in cornstarch and whisk until no more lumps.

7. Add the pasta with remaining liquid and cornstarch mixture to chicken and vegetables. Stir and cook over medium heat for a few minutes or until the sauce thickens.
8. To serve, sprinkle with grated parmesan cheese. Garnish with chopped parsley (optional garnish).

CHAPTER 8: BREAKFAST RECIPES

Oatmeal and Fruit Muffins

INGREDIENTS

- 1 1/2 cup whole wheat bread flour or all-purpose
- 1 cup quick-cooking oatmeal
- 3/4 cups brown sugar whole or dark
- 2 teaspoons baking powder
- 1/2 teaspoon salt
- 1 cup sour cream 5% or 14%
- 2 teaspoons baking soda
- 1/2 cup canola oil
- 2 eggs
- 1 tablespoon vanilla extract
- 2 cups fresh or frozen fruit (blueberries, cherries, peaches, blackberries, strawberries, berries, etc.)

PREPARATION

1. Preheat the oven to 350 ° F. In a bowl, combine flour, oats, baking powder, and salt with a fork. Cut the fruit into 1 to 1.5 cm pieces if they are larger.

2. Meanwhile, mix the baking soda with the sour cream in a measuring cup of 2 cups. Allow it to swell.
3. With an electric mixer, mix oil with eggs and vanilla. Add the brown sugar and mix well. Add swollen sour cream and mix gently.
4. Gradually add dry ingredients to moist ingredients. Mix gently between each addition. Add the fruits and mix with a spoon.
5. Divide the dough into muffin pans covered with paper boxes. Bake the muffins in the oven for about 20 minutes.

Blueberry Pancakes

INGREDIENTS

- 2-3 cups of flour
- 2 teaspoons baking powder
- 3/4 cup flaked oatmeal
- 1/4 cup sugar
- 1 3/4 cup milk (more or less depending on taste)
- 2 eggs
- 20 grams of melted butter
- 1 tablespoon vanilla extract
- a pinch of salt
- Blueberries at ease

INSTRUCTIONS

1. Mix the flour, baking powder, oatmeal, pinch of salt, and sugar.
2. Add milk, egg yolks, melted butter, and vanilla extract.
3. Raise the egg whites to the point, and add them to the mixture in an envelope.
4. Cook in a pan and add the blueberries in each pancake.
5. Serve with maple honey.

Breakfast with Avena Copos

INGREDIENTS:

- 250 ml of milk (can be from a cow, soy, oatmeal, rice)
- 3 heaped tablespoons of oat flakes (You can buy them at Mercadona)
- 1 tablespoon honey, sugar, or cinnamon
- Half-grated apple
- 1 handful of raisins
- Half banana cut
- 1 handful of walnuts, date chips, figs (any dried fruit)

PREPARATION:

1. Put the milk in a saucepan with the oatmeal and simmer.
2. When it starts to boil, leave about 5 minutes (stir thoroughly so that it does not stick). Then after 5 minutes, let stand a few minutes with the fire off (it will be more fluffy).
3. Put in a bowl and add the sweetener that you want along with the apple, banana, and nuts.
4. You can take it both hot and cold.

NOTES:

You can take them if you want only with milk. It's more important to put the oatmeal flakes, and if we put more rich things, it is already a DELICIOUS AND HEALTHY BREAKFAST!

Banana Breakfast Pancakes

INGREDIENTS :

- ½ cup (63g.) of wheat flour.
- ½ cup (80g.) of flaked oatmeal.
- 2 small bananas (160g.) mashed.

- Two eggs (100g.).
- 1 cup (240g.) Ideal, 0% Fat, and evaporated milk.
- 2 tablespoons (30g.) Brown sugar.
- 1 tablespoon (6g.) of cinnamon.
- 1 teaspoon (5g.) of butter.

DIRECTIONS:

1. In a bowl, combine all ingredients, except butter.
2. In a pan over medium heat, place the butter and wait until it melts.
3. Pour ¼ cup of the mixture over the pan, and cook until it begins to bubble.
4. Turn the pancake and cook for 1 minute or until it browns on the other side.
5. Serve and enjoy.

Orange And Red Blueberry Cookies

INGREDIENTS:

- 4 T (360g) of oatmeal in fine flakes
- 2 T (250g without bone) dates
- 1 cheaped the vanilla powder
- 1 T (120g) dried cranberries
- 2 organic oranges (its juice and peel)
- sweet orange essence salt - optional
- 2 C mild oil (sunflower or almond) - optional

DIRECTIONS

1. Wash the oranges and grate them. Make the juice and reserve.
2. Crush the dates.

3. Put in the robot: oat flakes, dates, orange zest, vanilla, and a pinch of salt. Crush until it begins to stick, and dates have been chopped small.
4. Add the juice of the oranges and crush again to incorporate. (200ml at most, if you get a little less, nothing happens)
5. Now, add the blueberries and mash — just a little, just enough for some to chop and others not.
6. Remove the robot and put it in a bowl.
7. Add the oil, although this is optional. If you do not have or do not want to put the oil and the dough is moistened so much that you can form the cookies, then you can skip it.
8. Make the cookies and put on the dehydrator tray. They do not need to be on teflex sheet or baking paper. I leave them as-is for the air to circulate better and be done before. Set the first hour at 52°, and the following at 42°. They will be done in about 6 hours or so; after 4 hours, you can turn them around.

Tuna Spinach Sandwich

INGREDIENTS
- The quantity of ingredients is to your liking and preference.
- Integral bread
- fresh and well-washed spinach
- tuna in well-drained water
- a ripe but firm avocado
- salt and pepper

INSTRUCTIONS
1. The spinach already washed and dried the short in thin strips, the finest you can.
2. What I do to achieve these strips is, I arrange several spinach leaves on top of each other, I make a small roll, and with a very sharp knife, I am cutting, and thus, they are excellent.

3. Avocado cut it into tiny cubes.
4. The bread is browned in a Teflon pan, on one side only.
5. Mix spinach with tuna and avocado.
6. Season the mixture with salt and pepper.
7. You put the stuffing in the bread and go.
8. Enjoy this delight.

Grilled eggplants with garlic and herbs

INGREDIENTS:

- 2 eggplants
- 1 teaspoon salt
- ½ cup extra virgin olive oil
- 3 grated garlic cloves
- 2 tablespoons chopped fresh parsley
- 2 tablespoons fresh oregano
- ½ teaspoon black pepper
- ½ extra teaspoon of salt

DIRECTIONS

1. Cut the eggplants into 5 mm slices and generously salt each of them. Let stand 15 minutes for the salt to extract moisture and bitterness from the eggplant. Clean each slice with a paper towel to remove excess moisture and salt.
2. Preheat the grill over medium heat.
3. On a large plate, mix olive oil, garlic, parsley, oregano, pepper, and salt. Pass each eggplant slice through the mixture so that it is covered with oil.
4. Roast about 6 minutes per side until golden brown and with grill marks. If they dry out, brush with more oil.
5. Serve with a drizzle of the remaining herbal oil.

Baked Oatmeal with Spiced Apple

INGREDIENTS

- one beaten egg
- 1/2 cup of applesauce
- 1 1/2 cup of milk 1% or nonfat
- 1 tsp of vanilla
- 2 tbsp of oil
- one chopped apple
- 2 cups of oats traditional
- 1 tsp of baking powder
- 1/4 teaspoon of salt
- 1 tsp of cinnamon

INGREDIENTS (from the top)

- 2 tbsp of brown sugar
- 2 tbsp of walnuts, chopped (optional)

PREPARATION

1. Heat the oven to 375° F.
2. Combine the egg, applesauce, milk, vanilla, and oil in a bowl. Enter the apple.
3. In another bowl, mix oats (rolled oats), baking powder, salt, and cinnamon. Add to liquid ingredients and mix well.
4. Pour the mixture into a ceramic baking plate and put it in the oven for 25 minutes.
5. Remove the bowl from the oven, sprinkle with brown sugar and nuts (optional) on top.
6. Return the bowl to the oven and cook for 3 to 4 minutes until the top is golden brown and the sugar bubbles.
7. Serve warm. Refrigerate leftovers within 2 hours.

Chicken and Pear Salad

INGREDIENTS

- Escarole, canons or watercress
- Grilled chicken
- Pear
- Pistachios
- sweet onion (rings)
- Pink pepper
- Pink salt
- Extra virgin olive oil 3 tablespoons
- 1 teaspoon Dijon mustard in grain
- 1 teaspoon honey

INSTRUCTIONS

1. Clean and cut delicious escarole or any other green leafy vegetable such as canons, watercress to which you add a few pieces of pear cut into segments or squares.
2. Add chopped pistachios.
3. You can use any other dried fruit that you like more or that you have in the pantry: pine nuts, pecans, almonds.
4. Peel and chop onion, which gives it a spicy point always.
5. And if you dare with the vinaigrette mix, a teaspoon of Dijon mustard in grain, a teaspoon of honey, extra virgin olive oil, lime juice and salt, and pink pepper.
6. Pink pepper is an ingredient that gives an extraordinary touch. In my opinion, you can crush some, and others, you leave them whole.
7. The so-called pink pepper, in reality, is the grain of a Brazilian pepper shaker. Its flavor is very peculiar, the mixture of sweet, citrus, little spicy flavor, and reminiscent of pine.
8. Finally, you add the roast chicken that you can buy well-packed or remains of some homemade preparation.

Spaghetti with broccoli sauce (broccoli) pesto type

INGREDIENTS:

- 500 gr. of spaghetti or noodles (use long pasta of your choice)
- 1 broccoli (broccoli) of approx. 600 gr.
- 2 tablespoons olive oil
- ½ medium onion
- 2 cloves of garlic
- 50 gr. of walnuts
- 1 cup chicken broth or vegetable broth
- 1 tablespoon of cream or sour cream or ½ cup of cream
- 50 gr. grated Parmesan cheese
- nutmeg to your liking
- salt and black pepper to your taste
- flaked chili or cayenne pepper to your liking (optional)

PREPARATION:

1. Wash and cut into broccoli (broccoli) on florets, making sure that the size is similar to cook at the same time. Cut across at the bottom of the trunk. This will make the trunk and the flower cook at the same time. Take advantage of the trunk, which is also very tasty. Peel it a bit and cut it into discs.
2. In a large pot with a lid, pour only two fingers of water. Add salt, mix well and introduce broccoli (broccoli). Try to place the florets with the trunk down and the flower up, since, in this way, the flower will not wilt during cooking. Cook covered over medium heat for 10 minutes or until a knife is easily inserted into the trunk.
3. Turn off the heat, drain the broccoli (broccoli) in a colander and return it to the pot.
4. While broccoli (broccoli) is cooking, cut the onion and garlic into brunoise and brown in a pan with a little olive oil until they are translucent. Turn off the heat, add the nuts and wait for the broccoli (broccoli) to be cooked.

5. Add the sautéed onion to broccoli (broccoli), and with the help of a crusher, blender, or blender, blend all the ingredients until you get a homogeneous mixture. Add chicken or vegetable broth, cream, nutmeg, salt, pepper and continue beating. Add grated Parmesan cheese and mix with the help of a spatula or wooden spoon. If you want it spicy, add some chili flakes to your liking.
6. Cover the pot and set aside until the pasta is cooked.
7. In a large pot with plenty of saltwater, cook the spaghetti or noodles following the manufacturer's instructions. Take care that you stay "al dente." Once prepared, save a ladle of spaghetti water and drain the remaining water.
8. Mix the spaghetti with the sauce and if you need more liquid, add some water that you reserved from the spaghetti.
9. Serve immediately and spread a little "Tomatina" sauce on top.

Quesadillas with Pears

INGREDIENTS

- 4 medium wheat whole wheat tortillas
- 1 cup of cheese grated (try cheddar or Jack)
- 1 cup of diced pears (fresh or canned and drained of liquid)
- 1/2 cup of chili green or red bell finely chopped
- 2 tbsp of onion, finely chopped (scallion, white or red)

PREPARATION

1. Divide the cheese, peas, chili peppers, and onions among the tortillas, covering almost half of each tortilla.
2. Heat a pan or iron over medium heat (300 degrees in an electric pan). Place one or two folded tortillas in a hot, dry pan until the cheese melts and the tortilla is browned lightly approximately 2-4 minutes.

3. With a large spatula, gently turn the quesadillas and cook the other side until they are a little golden, 2 to 4 minutes.
4. Put away to a plate and repeat until all tortillas are hot. Cut each cooked quesadilla in half and serve.
5. Refrigerate within the next 2 hours.

Notes

- Put the pears in cubes on paper towels for a couple of minutes to dry completely. This will help the quesadilla not be destroyed in the process!
- Do not have pears? Try fresh apples, grapes cut in half, or even cut bananas.
- To give more flavor: add finely cut cilantro, or use "pepper jack" type cheese.

Cranberry Quinoa Salad

INGREDIENTS

- 1 1/2 cups of water
- 1 cup raw quinoa, rinsed
- 1/4 cup chopped red pepper
- 1/4 cup yellow pepper, chopped
- 1 small red/purple onion, finely chopped
- 1 1/2 teaspoons curry powder
- 1/4 cup chopped fresh cilantro
- 1 lemon, juiced
- 1/4 cup toasted sliced almonds
- 1/2 cup chopped carrots
- 1/2 cup dried cranberries
- Salt and ground black pepper to taste.

INSTRUCTIONS

1. Pour the water into a saucepan and cover with a lid. Boil over high heat, then pour the quinoa, recover, and continue

over low heat until the water is absorbed, taking about 15 to 20 minutes. Transfer to a mixing bowl and chill in the refrigerator until cold.

2. Once cold, add the red pepper, yellow pepper, onion, curry powder, cilantro, lemon juice, sliced almonds, carrots, and blueberries. Season to taste with salt and pepper. Relax before serving

Winter fruit salad with lemon and poppy vinaigrette

INGREDIENTS

Vinaigrette

- ½ t. (125 mL) sugar
- 2 tbsp. (10 mL) onion, finely chopped
- ½ c. (2 mL) salt
- ⅓ t. (75 mL) lemon juice
- 1 C. (5 mL) Dijon mustard
- ⅔ cup (150 mL) vegetable oil
- 1 C. (15 mL) poppy seeds

Salad

- 1 large romaine lettuce apple, shredded into small pieces (about 10 t./2.5 L)
- 1 t. (250 mL) Swiss cheese, grated
- 1 t. (250 mL) cashews
- ¼ t. (50 mL) sweetened dehydrated cranberries
- 1 medium apple (1 t./250 mL)
- 1 medium pear (1 t./250 mL)

DIRECTIONS

1. In a blender or food processor, place sugar, onion, salt, lemon juice, and mustard. Put the lid on and mix until homogeneous.
2. While the machine is running, add the net oil slowly and stably, and mix until smooth and thick. Add the poppy seeds and mix for a few more seconds.
3. In a bowl, mix all the ingredients of the salad.

Salad in balsamic tempeh pot, strawberries, and cucumber

INGREDIENTS:

- 240g. of tempeh nature *
- 1/4 cup of tamari
- 1/4 cup of maple syrup *
- 1/4 cup of water
- 1/4 cup of balsamic vinegar
- 1 French shallot * finely chopped
- 1/3 cup of nutritional yeast
- 1 tbsp. mustard dijon
- 1 tbsp. vegetable oil table
- 1 c. olive oil
- 1/3 cup lemon juice
- 1 cup strawberries * diced
- 1 cup English cucumber * diced
- 2 cups red lettuce * coarsely chopped
- 1/3 cup ground seeds grilled pumpkin
- Salt and pepper

PREPARATION:

1. In a cauldron filled with boiling water, cook the tempeh for ten minutes. Drain and let stand for 1 to 2 minutes. Cut the boiled tempeh block into cubes and set aside.

2. In a bowl, add tamari, maple syrup, water, balsamic vinegar, French shallot, nutritional yeast, and Dijon mustard. Mix and reserve.
3. In a skillet over medium heat, add the vegetable oil and color the cubes of tempeh. Once lightly browned, pour all the ingredients from your bowl onto the cubes, then bring to a boil by raising the temperature of the pan to medium/high. Mix from time to time until all the liquid has evaporated — Reserve in a bowl.
4. In 2 Mason jars, divide olive oil and lemon juice equitably. Salt and pepper. Assemble the pots in equal portions and steps, adding diced strawberries, English cucumber cubes, tempeh cubes, leaf lettuce leaves, and roasted pumpkin seeds.
5. Store the Mason jars in the fridge and hang them with you in your lunches, in the park, or just for a quick meal on the way home from work. Turn the pot upside down, pour it into a bowl, mix, and enjoy immediately.

Lunch Recipes

Fish in tomato sauce

INGREDIENTS

- 4 frozen white fish fillets of your choice
- 2 cups cherry tomatoes cut in half
- 2 finely sliced garlic cloves
- 120 ml light chicken broth
- 60 ml of dry white wine (or use more chicken stock)
- 1/2 teaspoon salt
- 1/2 teaspoon black pepper
- 1/4 cup finely chopped fresh basil leaves (to garnish)

PREPARATION

1. Place the tomatoes, garlic, salt, and pepper in a pan over medium heat. Cook for 5 minutes or until tomatoes are soft.
2. Add chicken broth, white wine (if used), frozen fish fillets, and chopped basil. Cover and simmer for 20-25 minutes, until the fish is cooked.
3. Finally, sprinkle with an additional handful of chopped basil and serve on a bed of rice, couscous or quinoa, if desired.

Note: Thick white fish fillets such as cod, halibut, catfish, or mahi-mahi work best for this recipe.

Sea Bass and Peppers Salad

INGREDIENTS

- Very clean Seabass: A fillet of 150g.
- Assorted lettuces: 100g.
- Chives: To taste
- Fresh or roasted red pepper: 1
- Cherry tomatoes To taste
- Garlic clove and parsley 1
- Leek 1
- Carrot 1
- Olive oil One tablespoon
- Salt and lemon to taste

DIRECTIONS

1. We put the fillet of sea bass in aluminum foil. In the mortar, chop the garlic and parsley, add two small teaspoons of oil and cover the fillet of sea bass with it.
2. We also put some leek and carrot strips on the sea bass fillet (the vegetable ribbons can be made with the fruit peeler) and a little salt. Now, we close the foil tightly and take it into the oven at 120ºC for 8-10 minutes. Once cooked, let it cool.

3. In a salad bowl, put the lettuce mixture and chop the chives and pepper very finely. Then add it too. Add the cherry tomatoes cut into quarters. Add only a small teaspoon of olive oil, salt, and lemon as a dressing and stir well. Now, add the fish with the cooked vegetables and be ready to eat.

Mexican baked beans and rice

INGREDIENTS

- 5 ml (1 teaspoon) unsalted butter
- 1 chopped yellow onion
- 3/4 cup (190 mL) basmati rice
- 5 ml (1 teaspoon) ground cumin
- 1 seeded jalapeño pepper
- 300 ml (1 1/4 cups) chicken stock
- 125 ml (1/2 cup) tomato sauce
- 3/4 cup (190 mL) canned black kidney beans
- 30 ml (2 tablespoons) finely chopped parsley
- 1 lime
- Salt and pepper, to taste

PREPARATION

1. In a saucepan, melt the butter and add the onion. Simmer.
2. Add the rice and ground cumin. Continue cooking for about 2 minutes. Add the Jalapeno pepper. Deglaze with chicken stock and season.
3. Add the tomato sauce — cover and cook over medium heat for about 12 minutes.
4. When the rice is cooked, add the black beans and parsley. Continue cooking for minutes.
5. Add lime juice, salt, pepper, and serve.

Easy Baked Shepherd Pie

INGREDIENTS

- 500 grams of freshly ground duck meat
- 3 tablespoons oil or olive oil
- 1 small onion, finely chopped
- 1 tsp ready-made garlic and salt seasoning
- 1 tablespoon dry spice chimichurri
- 4 medium cooked and mashed potatoes
- 1 tablespoon full of butter
- 100 ml of milk
- 25 grams of grated Parmesan cheese
- 1 pinch of salt

PREPARATION

1. In a pan heat oil, onion, and fry.
2. Add the meat and garlic and salt seasoning.
3. Fry well until the accumulated meat water dries.
4. After the meat is fried, add enough water to cover the meat.
5. Let it cook with the pan without a lid until the water almost dries again.
6. Add the chimichurri, stir, and cook until the water dries, and allow the meat to fry until it's well dried.
7. Put the meat in an ovenproof dish and set aside.
8. Prepare a mash by mixing the remaining ingredients and spread over the meat.
9. Bake for about 20 minutes or until flushed.
10.   Remove and serve.

Fish in the herb, garlic, and tomato sauce

INGREDIENTS

- 6 teeth garlic peeled and whole
- 300 grams of halved mini onion

- 300 grams of halved pear (or cherry) tomato
- 1 packet of herbs (basil, parsley, and thyme) coarsely chopped
- 1/2 cup of olive oil
- 1 merluza fillet
- 2 cups wheat flour
- 3 egg
- 3 cups cornmeal
- black pepper to taste
- frying oil
- salt to taste

PREPARATION

1. In a large baking dish, place the garlic, onion, tomato, and herbs. Mix the olive oil, salt, and pepper.
2. Wrap the fish fillets and cover them with plastic wrap.
3. Refrigerate and marinate for 1 hour.
4. Remove the fish fillets, pass in the flour, then in the eggs beaten with a little salt and last in the cornmeal. Then refrigerate.
5. Put the baking sheet with the marinade in the oven, preheat to 200° C, and let it bake for about 20 minutes.
6. Remove the breaded fillets from the refrigerator and fry in hot oil until golden brown.
7. Serve the fish with the sauce in the baking dish.

Hot Salad with Kale and White Beans

INGREDIENTS:

- 1 large bunch of kale well washed
- 1-2 tablespoons olive oil
- 1 stem of fresh rosemary, with the leaves removed from the stem and cut

- 1 small onion, cut
- 1 large carrot, sliced
- ½ teaspoon finely grated lemon zest
- 1 clove garlic, minced
- Salt to taste
- 2 cups cooked lima beans or other white beans plus cooking broth or 1 can (14 ounces)
- 1 cup plain parsley, cut
- Extra virgin olive oil, to spray
- Juice from ½ to small lemon, to spray (optional)

PREPARATION

1. Remove the leaves from the kale stalks. Cut into bite-sized pieces. Set aside.
2. Drain the white beans, reserving their broth. If you use canned beans, drain and wash. Set aside.
3. In a large pot, heat the oil over medium-high heat until it starts to boil. Add the rosemary, reserving a teaspoon, let it boil for a moment, and then add the chopped onion, carrot, and lemon zest. Mix well and reduce the temperature. Cover and "sweat" the vegetables for minutes, or until they are soft and the onion is a little golden. Then stir occasionally to make sure they do not stick or burn.
4. Increase the temperature to medium-high. Add the cut garlic, stir and cook for 5 minutes. Add the cut greens with a good pinch of salt and sauté until they begin to wilt and soften.
5. Add ½ cup of the bean or water broth. Bring to a boil, lower the temperature for 10 to 15 minutes, or until the greens are soft, and the liquid has evaporated. Put a little more broth or water if the vegetables seem very dry.
6. Mix the chopped parsley and the remaining teaspoon of rosemary, cook for 1 minute, then add the beans to the pot. Mix carefully with the greens. Try the seasoning.

7. Put off the burner and let the quinoa stand covered for 5 minutes. Serve sprinkled with a little olive oil and some lemon juice.

Scallion Swordfish

INGREDIENTS

- 800 g of swordfish
- 1 lemon (medium)
- 1 dl of olive oil
- 2 Onions
- 1 dl of White Wine
- 1 c. (dessert) chopped parsley
- 4 royal gala apples
- 1 c. (soup) Butter
- 150 g chives
- Salt q.s.
- Paprika q.s.
- Salsa q.s.

PREPARATION

1. Season the swordfish slices with salt and lemon juice. Let them marinate for 30 minutes. After this time, fry them in olive oil. Add the peeled and sliced onions to half-moons and let them sauté.
2. Cool with white wine and season with a little more salt. Sprinkle with chopped parsley. Peel the apples cut them into wedges and sauté them in butter. Peel the spring onions and add them to the fruit.
3. Season with some salt and paprika. Serve the fish topped with the spring onions and accompanied with the sauteed apple and spring onions. Garnish with parsley.

Jambalaya Rice Recipe (also simply called Jambalaya)

INGREDIENTS

- 2 cups of needled rice
- 200g boneless, skinless chicken meat, diced
- 200g of thinly diced ham
- 1 medium onion, finely chopped
- 2 cloves garlic, minced
- 4 peeled, seedless tomatoes, chopped
- 1 stalk of chopped celery
- 1/2 diced red bell pepper
- 4 teaspoon chicken or shrimp background
- 2 tbsp tomato extract
- 2 tbsp butter
- 1/2 cup chopped green onions
- QB of salt
- 350 g of clean gray shrimp
- 1 lemon
- QB of freshly ground black pepper

Homemade Cajun Seasoning to taste

- 1 tsp garlic powder
- 1 tablespoon onion powder
- 1 tsp white ground pepper
- 1 tsp ground black pepper
- 1 teaspoon dried pepperoni pepper
- 1 tablespoon dry thyme
- 1 tablespoon dried oregano
- 1 tbsp spicy paprika
- 1 tablespoon dried tarragon
- 1 teaspoon ground cinnamon
- 1 teaspoon chili powder
- 1 tablespoon salt

- PS: add all ingredients and process or mash in the pestle.

PREPARATION

1. Season the prawns with lemon juice, salt, and ground pepper. Let it taste for 30 minutes. Then reserve
2. In a pan, melt the butter with a little olive oil and brown the chicken cubes. Reserve
3. In the pan, fat sauté the onion and garlic until it withers.
4. Add celery, peppers, and tomatoes, and sauté for 2 minutes.
5. Add the rice and sauté; Add tomato extract and chicken or shrimp background.
6. Mix well and add the homemade Cajun spice to taste; Cook for 15 minutes over low heat, then cover without stirring.
7. Add the reserved shrimp and cook another 5 minutes or until it's well-dried. Then mix slightly.
8. Remove from heat, sprinkle with green onions and serve very hot

Chick Curry (Thai Chicken)

INGREDIENTS

- 2 skinless, boneless chicken breasts (not too small)
- 3 tablespoons olive oil
- 1 small onion, finely chopped
- 2 cloves garlic, minced
- 3 tablespoons curry powder
- 1 teaspoon ground cinnamon
- 1 teaspoon paprika
- 1 bay leaf
- 1/2 teaspoon freshly grated ginger root
- 1 tbsp tomato extract
- 1 bottle of coconut milk
- 1/2 lemon (juice)

- 1 red bell pepper
- 1 cup pineapple (optional)

PREPARATION

1. In a bowl season the chicken cubes with salt and lemon juice and set aside.
2. Put the olive oil, garlic, onion, and saute in a pan until golden brown.
3. Then put the chicken in the pan and saute until golden brown.
4. Add pineapple (optional), curry, cinnamon, paprika, bay leaf, tomato extract, ginger, and red pepper. Saute for a few more minutes (if necessary, add a cup of water).
5. Add coconut milk, cook for a few more minutes and serve.

Fried breaded lasagna with marinara sauce

INGREDIENTS

- 6 large slices of lasagna
- 1 cup of ricotta or cottage cheese
- 1 cup of mozzarella cheese
- 3 eggs
- ½ tablespoon of Italian seasoning
- 1 tablespoon of chopped parsley
- 1 clove of crushed garlic
- salt and pepper
- ¼ cup wheat flour
- c / n breadcrumbs
- c / n vegetable oil

DIRECTIONS

1. Cook in a large saucepan with water before the lasagna, according to the manufacturer's instructions.
2. Place the lasagna sheets on a previously greased baking sheet.
3. Combine ricotta cheese, mozzarella cheese, 1 egg, Italian seasoning, parsley, garlic and salt, and pepper to taste in a bowl. Incorporate all ingredients very well.
4. Distribute the previous mixture on each of the lasagna sheets and roll very well by pressing the filling.
5. To breach, pass each lasagna roll through bowls of flour, bowl with 2 beaten eggs, and to finish the dish with the breadcrumbs. Then enter the freezer for 30 minutes.
6. Heat plenty of oil in a deep pan. Introduce the lasagna rolls one by one and fry for 2 to 3 minutes. Place on the paper towel to remove excess oil.
7. Cut lasagna rolls in half, and serve on a marinara sauce base.

Marinara sauce:

1. In a medium saucepan heat two tablespoons of oil, add 1 finely chopped onion and 1 clove of crushed garlic and brown for 5 minutes.
2. Stir with a wooden spoon to prevent burning. Add 2 cups of chopped tomato, two tablespoons of tomato paste, and 2 tablespoons of chopped fresh basil, ½ tablespoon of ground black pepper, 1 teaspoon of ground oregano and ½ tablespoon of salt.
3. Cook until the sauce boils. Put it on low heat and continue cooking for 20 minutes or until the sauce acquires a thick consistency.

Baked Mushrooms with Pumpkin And Chipotle Polenta

INGREDIENTS

- 900 g mix of mushrooms, such as maitake, jasmine ear and black shimeji - coarsely chopped - thinly sliced porcini crimini mushrooms - and coarsely chopped shiitakessem stalks
- About 1/3 cup of extra virgin olive oil
- 1 garlic head, crushed cloves
- A small handful of sage, finely chopped or sliced
- Sea salt and freshly ground black pepper.
- 1 cup cooked pumpkin puree
- 3 cups chicken broth
- Nutmeg, freshly grated
- 1 chipotle adobo sauce, seedless and finely chopped, plus a small spoon of adobo sauce
- 1 cup quick-cooking polenta
- 2 tbsp butter
- 2 tbsp honey
- Roasted seeds for decoration
- Chives, minced, for decoration

PREPARATION

1. Preheat the oven to 220 ºC.
2. Mix the mushrooms with extra virgin olive oil, garlic, brine, salt, and pepper and bake for 25 minutes.
3. Meanwhile, in a small pan, put it pumpkin puree over medium heat, along with some chicken broth to dilute.
4. Season with salt, pepper, and nutmeg.
5. In another pan, put the remaining stock and bring to a boil, then add the chipotle, adobo sauce, polenta and mix using a wire whisk. Continue beating the polenta until the sides are far from the pan walls, then add the butter, honey, and then beat again.
6. Combine pumpkin and polenta and serve in individual shallow bowls.
7. Top with roasted mushrooms and Siva with roasted seeds and chives for garnish.

Dinner Recipes

Meat and Kidney Pie

INGREDIENTS

- 500g beef (diced)
- 225g kidneys (cow or veal, heavy clean and cut)
- 1 onion (chopped)
- 150g mushrooms (clean and sliced)
- 250 ml beef broth
- 2 tbsp. tomato paste (optional)
- 1 tbsp. cornstarch
- 250g puff pastry (or broken dough)
- 1 egg (beaten)
- 1 tsp. salt
- 1 tsp. pepper (ground black pepper)
- 3 tbsp. oil
- water (to dissolve cornstarch)

INSTRUCTIONS

1. Heat the oil in a casserole and brown the beef. We take it out and reserve it.
2. In the same oil, we fry the onion until it softens.
3. Add the kidneys, tomato paste, if used, mushrooms, and broth.
4. Cover the casserole and lower the heat when the sauce begins to boil, letting it simmer until the meat is tender about 30 minutes.
5. When it's almost done, we can start heating the oven at 180º C.

6. Mix the cornstarch with a little water and add it to the casserole where the meat and kidneys are being cooked, mix with the sauce, season with salt and pepper, and let the stew cook for five more minutes, until the sauce thickens.
7. Pass the meat and kidneys with their sauce to a baking dish.
8. Then stretch the dough enough to cover the source as a cover. Also, moisten the edge of the fountain with water and press the dough against the edge to seal it.
9. Cut in the middle so that the steam can escape, and then paint the dough with a beaten egg.
10. Put the meat and kidney pie in the oven and let it be done for 30 minutes, or until the dough that covers the cake is browned.
11. Lastly, serve the cake very hot almost as soon as it comes out of the oven so that the steam does not soften the dough.

Cauliflower and Pumpkin Casserole

INGREDIENTS

- 2 tbsp. olive oil
- 1/4 medium of yellow onion, minced
- 6 cups of chopped forage kale into small pieces (about 140g)
- 1 little of clove garlic, minced
- Salt and freshly ground black pepper
- 1/2 cup of low sodium chicken broth
- 2 cups of 1.5 cm diced pumpkin (about 230 g)
- 2 cups of 1.5 cm diced zucchini (about 230 g)
- 2 tbsp. mayonnaise
- 3 cups frozen, thawed brown rice
- 1 cup grated Swiss cheese
- 1/3 cup of grated Parmesan
- 1 cup of panko flour
- 1 large beaten egg

- Cooking spray

PREPARATION

1. Preheat oven to 200° C. Heats the oil in a large nonstick skillet over medium heat. Add onions and cook, occasionally stirring, until browned and tender (about 5 minutes). Add the cabbage, garlic, and 1/2 teaspoon salt and 1/2 teaspoon pepper and cook until the cabbage is light (about 2 minutes).
2. Add the stock and continue to cook until the cabbage withers, and most of the stock evaporates (about 5 minutes). Add squash, zucchini, and 1/2 teaspoon salt and mix well. Continue cooking until the pumpkin begins to soften (about 8 minutes). Remove from heat and add mayonnaise.
3. In a bowl, combine cooked vegetables, brown rice, cheese, 1/2 cup flour, and large egg and mix well. Spray a 2-liter casserole with cooking spray. Spread the mixture across the bottom of the pan and cover with the remaining flour, 1/4 teaspoon salt and a few pinches of pepper. Bake until the squash and zucchini are tender and the top golden and crispy (about 35 minutes). Serve hot.

Advance Preparation Tip: Freeze the casserole for up to 2 weeks. Cover with aluminum foil and heat at 180 ° C until warm (35 to 45 minutes).

Thai beef salad Tears of the Tiger

INGREDIENTS

- 800g of beef tenderloin
- For the marinade :
- 2 tablespoons of soy sauce
- 1 tablespoon soup of honey
- 1 pinch of the pepper mill
- For the sauce :

- 1 small bunch of fresh coriander
- 1 small bouquet of mint
- 3 tablespoons soup of fish sauce
- lemon green
- 1 clove of garlic
- tablespoons soup of sugar palm (or brown sugar)
- 1 bird pepper or ten drops of Tabasco
- 1 small glass of   raw Thai rice to make grilled rice powder
- 200 g of arugula or young shoots of salad

PREPARATION

1. Cut the beef tenderloin into strips and put it in a container. Sprinkle with 2 tablespoons soy sauce, 1 tablespoon honey, and pepper. Although soak thoroughly and let marinate 1 hour at room temperature.
2. Meanwhile, prepare the roasted rice powder. Pour a glass of Thai rice into an anti-adhesive pan. Dry color the rice, constantly stirring to avoid burning. When it has a lovely color, get rid of it on a plate and let it cool.
3. When it has cooled, reduce it to powder by mixing it with the robot.
4. Wash and finely chop mint and coriander. Put in a container and add lime juice, chopped garlic clove, 3 tablespoons Nuoc mam, 3 tablespoons brown sugar, 3 tablespoons water, 1 tablespoon sauce soy, and a dozen drops of Tabasco. Mix well and let stand the time that the sugar melts and the flavors mix.
5. Place a bed of salad on a dish. Cook the beef strips put them on the salad. Sprinkle with the spoonful of sauce and roasted rice powder. To be served as is or with a Thai cooked white rice scented.

Stuffed apples with shrimp

INGREDIENTS

- 6 medium apples
- 1 lemon juice
- 2 tablespoons butter

Filling:

- 300g of shrimp
- 1 onion minced
- ½ cup chopped parsley
- 2 tbsp flour
- 1 can of cream/cream
- 100g of curd
- 1 tablespoon butter
- 1 tbsp pepper sauce
- Salt to taste

PREPARATION

1. Cut a cap from each apple, remove the seeds a little from the pulp on the sides, and put the pulp in the bottom, but leaving a cavity.
2. Pass a little lemon and some butter on the apples, bake them in the oven. Remove from oven, let cool and bring to freeze.
3. Prepare the shrimp sauce in a pan by mixing the butter with the flour, onion, parsley, and pepper sauce.
4. Then add the prawn shrimp to the sauce. When boiling, mix the cream cheese and sour cream.
5. Stuff each apple. Serve hot or cold, as you prefer.

A Quick Recipe of Grilled Chicken Salad with Oranges

INGREDIENTS:

- 75 ml (1/3 cup) orange juice
- 30 ml (2 tablespoons) lemon juice
- 45 ml (3 tablespoons) of extra virgin olive oil
- 15 ml (1 tablespoon) Dijon mustard
- 2 cloves of garlic, chopped
- 1 ml (1/4 teaspoon) salt, or as you like
- Freshly ground pepper to your taste
- 1 lb. (450g) skinless chicken breast, trimmed
- 25g (1/4 cup) pistachio or flaked almonds, toasted
- 600g (8c / 5 oz) of mesclun, rinsed and dried
- 75g (1/2 cup) minced red onion
- 2 medium oranges, peeled, quartered and sliced

PREPARATION:

1. Place the orange juice, lemon juice, oil, mustard, garlic, salt, and pepper in a small bowl or jar with an airtight lid; whip or shake to mix. Reserve 75 milliliters (1/3 cup) of this salad vinaigrette and 45 milliliters (three tablespoons) for basting.
2. Place the rest of the vinaigrette in a shallow glass dish or resealable plastic bag. Add the chicken and turn it over to coat. Cover or close and marinate in the refrigerator for at least 20 minutes or up to two hours.
3. Preheat the barbecue over medium heat. Lightly oil the grill by rubbing it with a crumpled paper towel soaked in oil (use the tongs to hold the paper towel). Remove the chicken from the marinade and discard the marinade. Grill the chicken 10 to 15 centimeters (four to six inches) from the heat source, basting the cooked sides with the basting vinaigrette until it is no longer pink in the center, and Instant-read thermometer inserted in the thickest part records 75° C (170° F). Do this for four to six minutes on each side. Transfer the chicken to a cutting board and let it rest for five minutes.
4. Meanwhile, grill almonds (or pistachios) in a small, dry pan on medium-low heat, stirring constantly, until lightly

browned, about two to three minutes. Transfer them to a bowl and let them cool.

5. Place the salad and onion mixture in a large bowl. Mix with the vinaigrette reserved for the salad. Divide the salad into four plates. Slice chicken and spread on salads. Sprinkle orange slices on top and sprinkle with pistachios (or almonds).

Red Curry with Vegetable

INGREDIENTS

- 600g sweet potatoes
- 200g canned chickpeas
- 2 leek whites
- 2 tomatoes
- 100g of spinach shoots
- 40 cl of coconut milk
- 1 jar of Greek yogurt
- 1 lime
- 3 cm fresh ginger
- 1 small bunch of coriander
- 1/2 red onion
- 2 cloves garlic
- 4 tbsp. red curry paste
- salt

PREPARATION

1. Peel the sweet potatoes and cut them into pieces. Clean the leek whites and cut them into slices. Peel and seed the tomatoes.
2. Mix the Greek yogurt with a drizzle of lime juice, chopped onion, salt, and half of the coriander leaves.

3. In a frying pan, heat 15 cl of coconut milk until it reduces and forms a multitude of small bubbles. Brown curry paste with chopped ginger and garlic.
4. Add vegetables, drained chickpeas, remaining coconut milk, and salt. Cook for 20 min covered, then 5 min without lid for the sauce to thicken.
5. When serving, add spinach sprouts and remaining coriander. Serve with the yogurt sauce.

Baked Turkey Breast With Cranberry Sauce

INGREDIENTS

- 2 kilos of whole turkey breast
- 1 tablespoon olive oil
- 1/4 cup onion
- 2 cloves of garlic
- thyme
- poultry seasonings
- you saved
- coarse-grained salt
- 2 butter spoons
- 1/4 cup minced echallot
- 1/4 cup chopped onion
- 1 clove garlic
- 2 tablespoons flour
- 1 1/2 cups of blueberries
- 2 cups apple cider
- 2 tablespoons maple honey
- peppers

PREPARATION

1. Grind in the blender ¼ cup onion, 2 garlic with herbs. Add 1 tablespoon of oil and spread the breast with this.

2. Put in the baking tray, add a cup of citron and bake at 350 Fahrenheit (180 ° C) to have a thermometer record 165 Fahrenheit (75 ° C) inside, about an hour, add ½ cup of water if necessary.
3. Bring the citron to a boil, add the blueberries, and leave a few minutes. In the butter (2 tablespoons), acitronar the onion (1/4 cup), echallot, and garlic (1 clove).
4. Add the flour to the onion and echallot and leave a few minutes. Add the citron, cranberries, and honey and leave on low heat. Season with salt and pepper, let the blueberries are soft, go to the processor, and if you want to strain.
5. Return to the fire and let it thicken slightly.
6. Slice the thin turkey breast and serve with the blueberry sauce.

Parsnip soup, pear with smoked nuts

INGREDIENTS

For the soup:

500g of chopped parsnips, 1 tablespoon of olive oil, 4 sprigs of thyme, salt and pepper, 1 chopped onion, 1 tablespoon of margarine, 2 peeled and chopped pears, 800 ml of vegetable stock, 600 ml of milk, 75g of crushed California Nuts until a flour texture is achieved

For smoked nuts:

2 tsp of maple syrup, 1 teaspoon of smoked paprika, 2 teaspoons of soy sauce, 50 g of California Nuts, 1 tablespoon of chopped scallions and a dash of olive oil to decorate it.

DIRECTION

1. Preheat the oven to 180ºC. Place the parsnips on a baking sheet and squirt olive oil. Season with thyme, pepper, and salt mix well and bake for 25-30 minutes until golden brown.

2. Meanwhile, prepare smoked nuts. Mix the maple syrup, paprika, and soy sauce, spread on the nuts, and mix well. Position the nuts on a baking sheet and bake them for 8-10 minutes. Remove from the oven and let cool.
3. Next, sauté the onion with the margarine over medium heat. Add the pear and continue skipping for 8-10 more minutes.
4. Add the parsnip and the vegetable stock to the pan and continue cooking for 15 more minutes with the lid on. Add the milk and stir until creamy. Add the crushed nuts and season to taste.
5. Place the soup in bowls and decorate with smoked nuts and chopped chives. Add a dash of olive oil and serve.

Moroccan style chickpea soup

INGREDIENTS

- 4 ripe tomatoes, chopped
- 250g of cooked chickpeas.
- 1 chopped onion.
- 1 branch of chopped celery.
- 2 chicken thighs
- 2 tablespoons chopped fresh cilantro.
- 2 tablespoons chopped fresh parsley.
- 1 tablespoon turmeric.
- 1 tablespoon of cinnamon coffee
- 2 tablespoons grated fresh ginger coffee.
- A few strands of saffron.
- 4 tablespoons olive oil.
- A nip of sea salt and black pepper.
- Half grated zucchini with spiralizer (noodle substitute).

PREPARATION

1. We marinate chicken thighs with cinnamon and turmeric.

2. In a deep casserole, sauté chicken thighs in olive oil and brown them for about 3-4 minutes.
3. Then add the chopped onion and grated ginger. We stir well.
4. Add the celery, parsley, and cilantro. Saute the whole over medium heat for a few minutes.
5. Next, we remove the chicken thighs and reserve them.
6. Add the chopped tomatoes and a tablespoon of olive oil to the casserole.
7. In a cup of hot water, we soak the saffron threads. Then add the saffron along with the water to the casserole.
8. Then add the chicken and three more cups of hot water.
9. Add the salt and pepper.
10.   Cover the casserole and let the whole cook for half an hour, stirring occasionally.
11.   Remove the chicken from the casserole, remove the bones, and add the shredded meat back to the casserole.
12.   Finally, we incorporate the chickpeas.
13.   Prepare the "spaghetti" zucchini with the spiralizer (noodle substitutes).
14.   We serve the soup in bowls, incorporating the zucchini spaghetti on top.

Tuscan soup of chard and white beans

INGREDIENTS

- 2 slices of finely chopped bacon
- 1 chopped onion
- 1 clove garlic minced
- 1/4 c. nutmeg (optional)
- 1/8 c. hot pepper flakes (optional)
- 6-7 cups chicken broth, or more as needed
- 1 can (540 ml) of white beans, drained and rinsed
- 2 tbsp. sun-dried tomatoes, chopped
- 1 piece of Parmesan rind (about 1/2 cup)

- 1 bunch of chard red or white
- 1/4 cup small pasta for soup
- 5 large sliced sage leaves
- 5 fresh basil leaves, chopped (optional)
- 1 C. grated Parmesan cheese, divided (optional)
- 1 C. extra virgin olive oil, divided (optional)

PREPARATION

1. In a big saucepan over medium heat, brown bacon with onion, garlic, nutmeg, and pepper flakes for 5 minutes. Add chicken broth and beans. Bring to a boil. Stir in the dried tomatoes and Parmesan rind. Reduce heat and cook for 10 minutes.
2. Meanwhile, seed Swiss chard and slice stems into 3/4 inch lengths. Cut the leaves into 1-inch wide strips. Add the stems and pasta to the soup. Reserve the leaves for later. Reduce to low heat and simmer gently until the pasta is tender about 10 minutes. Add Swiss chard and basil leaves and simmer for 3-4 minutes.
3. Transfer soup to bowls sprinkles with parmesan and drizzle with olive oil, if desired.

Desserts And Sweets

Oatmeal and berry muffins

INGREDIENTS

- 1 cup (250 mL) non-blanched all-purpose flour
- ½ cup (125 mL) quick-cooking oatmeal 1/2 cup
- (160 mL) stuffed brown sugar
- 1/2 tbsp (1/2 cup) tea) baking soda
- 2 eggs

- 125 ml (1/2 cup) applesauce
- 60 ml (1/4 cup)
- orange canola oil 1, grated rind only
- 1 lemon, grated rind
- 15 ml (1 tbsp) lemon juice
- 180 ml (3/4 cup) fresh raspberries (see note)
- 180 ml (3/4 cup) fresh or blueberries (or blackberries)

PREPARATION

1. Put the grill at the center of the oven. Preheat oven to 180° C (350° F). Line 12 muffin cups with paper or silicone trays.
2. In a bowl, combine flour, oatmeal, brown sugar, and baking soda. Book.
3. In a big bowl, whisk together eggs, applesauce, oil, citrus zest, and lemon juice. Add the dry ingredients to the wooden spoon. Add the berries and mix gently.
4. Spread the mixture in the boxes. Sprinkle top with pistachio muffins. Bake for 20 to 22 minutes or until a toothpick inserted in the center of a muffin comes out clean. Let cool.

Crunchy Blueberry and Apples

INGREDIENTS

Crunchy

- 1 cup (1¼ cup) quick-cooking oatmeal
- ¼ cup (60 mL) brown sugar
- ¼ cup (60 mL) unbleached all-purpose flour
- 90 ml (6 tablespoons) melted margarine

Garnish

- 125 ml (½ cup) brown sugar
- 20 ml (4 teaspoons) cornstarch
- 1 liter (4 cups) fresh or frozen blueberries (not thawed)

- 500 ml (2 cups) grated apples
- 1 Tbsp.
- (15 mL) melted margarine 15 mL (1 tablespoon) lemon juice

PREPARATION

1. Put the grill at the center of the oven. Preheat oven to 180 ° C (350 ° F).
2. In a bowl, mix dry ingredients. Add the margarine and mix until the mixture becomes moistened. Book.
3. In a 20-cm (8-inch) square baking pan, combine brown sugar and cornstarch. Add the fruits, margarine, lemon juice, and mix well. Cover with crisp and bake between 55 minutes and 1 hour, or until the crisp is golden brown. Serve warm or cold.

Raspberry feast meringue with cream diplomat

INGREDIENTS

Preparation of meringue

- 2 egg whites
- 1/2 cup caster sugar
- 1/4 tsp. vanilla extract
- 1/4 cup crumbled barley sugar

Raspberry mousse preparation

- 1 cup frozen raspberries
- 1/4 cup water
- 2 tbsp. Raspberry Jell-O Powder with No Added Sugar
- 1 1/2 cup Cool Whip
- 1 bowl fresh raspberries

PREPARATION

1. To make the meringue, preheat the oven to 350° F (175° C) and line a baking sheet with parchment paper.
2. In a blender or bowl, whisk egg whites until the foam is obtained. Gently add the sugar while whisking until you get firm, shiny picks. Stir in vanilla extract and crumbled barley sugar.
3. Shape the meringues on the coated cookie sheet and place in the preheated oven. Turn off the oven and wait 2 hours. Do not open the oven. Once the meringues are dry, break the meringues into small bites.
4. To make the mousse, put frozen raspberries and water in a small saucepan. Heat until raspberries melt and are tender. Put these raspberries in a blender. Add the Jell-O powder and mix. Once the raspberries have completely cooled, incorporate the Cool Whip.
5. To shape the raspberry, place in balloon glasses for individual portions or in a large cake pan first a layer of raspberry mousse, then a layer of meringue, then fresh raspberries. Repeat the layers. Refrigerate for a few hours before serving.

Cheesecake mousse with raspberries

INGREDIENTS

- 1 cup light lemonade filling
- 1 can 8 oz cream cheese at room temperature
- 3/4 cup SPLENDA no-calorie sweetener pellets
- 1 tbsp. at t. of lemon zest
- 1 tbsp. at t. vanilla extract
- 1 cup fresh or frozen raspberries

PREPARATION

1. Beat the cream cheese until it is sparkling; add 1/2 cup SPLENDA® Granules and mix until melted. Stir in lemon zest and vanilla.
2. Reserve some raspberries for decoration. Crush the rest of the raspberries with a fork and mix them with 1/4 cup SPLENDA pellets until they are melted.
3. Lightly add the lump and cheese filling, and then gently but quickly add crushed raspberries. Share this mousse in 6 ramekins with a spoon and keep in the refrigerator until tasting.
4. Garnish mousses with reserved raspberries and garnish with fresh mint before serving.

Almond Meringue Cookies

INGREDIENTS

- 2 egg whites or 4 tbsp. pasteurized egg whites (at room temperature)
- 1 Tbsp. tartar cream
- ½ tsp.
- ½ teaspoon almond extract vanilla extract
- ½ cup white sugar

PREPARATION

1. Preheat the oven to 300° F.
2. Whisk the egg whites with the cream of tartar until the volume has doubled. Add other ingredients and whip until peaks form.
3. Using two teaspoons, drop a spoonful of meringue onto parchment paper with the back of the other spoon.
4. Bake at 300° F for about 25 minutes or until the meringues are crisp. Place in an airtight container.

Fresh Cranberry Pie

INGREDIENTS

- 1 ½ cup crumbled Graham crackers
- ¼ cup salt-free chopped pecans
- 1 ¾ cup Splenda Sweetener
- ½ cup non-hydrogenated salt-free margarine
- 1 ½ cup freshly picked cranberries
- 2 egg whites
- 1 tbsp. thawed apple juice concentrate
- 1 tbsp. vanilla extract
- 1 liter Cool Whip Whipped Topping, thawed

Cranberry Frosting:

- ¼ cup Splenda Sweetener
- ¼ cup caster sugar
- 1 Tbsp. cornstarch
- ¾ cup fresh cranberries
- ¾ cup of water

PREPARATION

1. Preheat oven to 375 ° F (190 ° C).
2. Mix crumbled crackers, pecans, and ¾ cup of Splenda. Add the margarine, mix well, and arrange on a hinged mold pressing on the bottom and the sides. Bake dough for 6 minutes or until slightly browned. Then let it cool.
3. Mix the cranberries with 1 cup of Splenda. Let stand for 5 minutes. Add the egg whites, apple juice, and vanilla. Beat at low speed until foamy, and then beat at high speed for 5 to 8 minutes until mixture is firm.
4. Stir in the whipped topping in the cranberry mixture. Pour the mixture over the pre-cooked dough. Refrigerate, at least, 4 hours until the mixture is firm.

5. To make the icing, mix the sugar, Splenda, and cornstarch in a saucepan. Stir in cranberries and water. Cook, stir until bubbles appear. Continue cooking, occasionally stir until cranberry skin comes off. Use the mixture at room temperature. Do not refrigerate: the sauce may crystallize and become opaque.
6. Remove the tart from the pan and arrange on a serving platter, using a spoon, coat with icing.

Entries And Snacks

Eggplant and chickpea bites

INGREDIENTS

- 3 large aubergines cut in half (make a few cuts in the flesh with a knife) Spray
- oil
- 2 large cloves garlic, peeled and deglazed
- 2 tbsp. coriander powder
- 2 tbsp. cumin seeds
- 400g canned chickpeas, rinsed and drained
- 2 Tbsp. chickpea flour
- Zest and juice of 1/2 lemon
- 1/2 lemon quartered for serving
- 3 tbsp. tablespoon of polenta

PREPARATION

1. Heat the oven to 200ºC (180ºC rotating heat, gas level 6). Spray the eggplant halves generously with oil and place them on the meat side up on a baking sheet. Sprinkle with coriander and cumin seeds, and then place the cloves of garlic on the plate. Season and roast for 40 minutes until the

flesh of eggplant is completely tender. Reserve and let cool a little.

2. Scrape the flesh of the eggplant in a bowl with a spatula and throw the skins in the compost. Thoroughly scrape and make sure to incorporate spices and crushed roasted garlic. Add chickpeas, chickpea flour, zest, and lemon juice. Crush roughly and mix well, check to season. Do not worry if the mixture seems a bit soft - it will firm up in the fridge.

3. Form about twenty pellets and place them on a baking sheet covered with parchment paper. Let stand in the fridge for at least 30 minutes.

4. Preheat oven to 180ºC (rotating heat 160ºC, gas level 4). Remove the meatballs from the fridge and coat them by rolling them in the polenta. Place them back on the baking sheet and spray a little oil on each. Roast for 20 minutes until golden and crisp. Serve with lemon wedges. You can also serve these dumplings with a spicy yogurt dip with harissa, this delicious but spicy mashed paste of hot peppers and spices from the Maghreb.

Popcorn with sugar and spice

INGREDIENTS

- 8 cups hot popcorn
- 2 tablespoons unsalted butter
- 2 tablespoons sugar
- 1/2 teaspoon cinnamon
- 1/4 teaspoon nutmeg

PREPARATION

1. Popping the corn; put aside.
2. Heat the butter, sugar, cinnamon, and nutmeg in the microwave or saucepan over a range fire until the butter is melted and the sugar dissolved.

3. Be careful not to burn the butter.
4. Sprinkle the corn with the spicy butter, and mix well.
5. Serve immediately for optimal flavor.

Baba Ghanouj

INGREDIENTS

- 1 large aubergine, cut in half lengthwise
- 1 head of garlic, unpeeled
- 30 ml (2 tablespoons) of olive oil
- Lemon juice to taste

PREPARATION

1. Put the grill at the center of the oven. Preheat the oven to 350° F. Line a baking sheet with parchment paper.
2. Place the eggplant on the plate, skin side up. Roast until the meat becomes so tender and detaches easily from the skin. Do this for about 1 hour, depending on the size of the eggplant. Let cool.
3. Meanwhile, cut the tip of the garlic cloves. Place the garlic cloves in a square of aluminum foil. Fold the edges of the sheet and fold to form a tightly wrapped foil. Roast with the eggplant until tender, about 20 minutes. Let cool. Purée the pods with a garlic press.
4. With a spoon, scoop out the flesh of the eggplant and place it in the bowl of a food processor. Add the garlic puree, the oil, and the lemon juice. Stir until purée is smooth and pepper.
5. Serve with mini pita bread.

Baked pita chips

INGREDIENTS

- 3 pita loaves (6 inches)
- 3 tablespoons olive oil
- Chili powder

PREPARATION

1. Separate each bread in half with scissors, to obtain 6 round pieces. Cut each piece into eight points. Brush each with olive oil and sprinkle with chili powder. Bake at 350° F for about 15 minutes until crisp.

Mixes of snacks

INGREDIENTS

- 6 c. margarine
- 2 tbsp worcestershire sauce
- 1 ½ tbsp. spice salt
- ¾ c. garlic powder
- ½ tsp. onion powder
- 3 cups of Crispix
- 3 cups of Cheerios
- 3 cups of corn flakes
- 1 cup of Kix
- 1 cup of pretzels
- 1 cup of broken bagel chips into 1-inch pieces

PREPARATION

1. Preheat the oven to 250F (120C)
2. Melt the margarine in a large roasting pan. Stir in the seasoning. Gradually add the remaining ingredients by mixing so that the coating is uniform.
3. Cook 1 hour, stirring every 15 minutes. Spread on paper towels to let it cool. Store in a tightly-closed container.

Herbal Cream Cheese Tartines

INGREDIENTS

- 20 regular round melba crackers
- 1 clove garlic, halved
- 1 cup cream cheese spread
- ¼ cup chopped herbs such as chives, dill, parsley, tarragon or thyme
- 2 tbsp. minced French shallot or onion
- ½ tsp. black pepper
- 2 tbsp. tablespoons water

PREPARATION

1. In a medium-sized bowl, combine the cream cheese, herbs, shallot, pepper, and water with a hand blender.
2. Rub the crackers with the cut side of the garlic clove.
3. Serve the cream cheese with the rusks

Spicy crab dip

INGREDIENTS

- 1 can of 8 oz softened cream cheese
- 1 tbsp. to s. finely chopped onions
- 1 tbsp. at t. lemon juice
- 2 tbsp. at t. Worcestershire sauce
- 1/8 tsp. at t. black
- pepper Cayenne pepper to taste
- 2 tbsp. to s. of milk or non-fortified rice drink
- 1 can of 6 oz of crabmeat

PREPARATION

1. Preheat the oven to 375° F (190° C).
2. Pour the cream cheese into a bowl. Add the onions, lemon juice, Worcestershire sauce, black pepper, and cayenne pepper. Mix well. Stir in the milk/rice drink. Add the crabmeat and mix until you obtain a homogeneous mixture.
3. Pour the mixture into a baking dish. Cook without covering for 15 minutes or until bubbles appear. Serve hot with low-sodium crackers or triangle cut pita bread. OR
4. Microwave until bubbles appear, about 4 minutes, then stir every 1 to 2 minutes.

Part 2

Chapter One Introduction To Renal Diet

How do the kidneys work?

Depending on body weight, 4 to 6 liters of blood circulates in the body. Blood is transported to the kidneys through the renal arteries. Every day, about 1,500 liters of blood pass through the kidneys, which are purified by the work of about a million nephrons.

Nephrons consist of small filters called glomeruli that separate water, salts, and impurities from the blood. Protein and blood cells remain in it. The filtered fluid (primary urine) is transported through small channels. There are cells of a particular type (tubular cells) that cause water and salts such as sodium, calcium, phosphorus, and magnesium to return to the blood. The remainder of the fluid is excreted as ultimate urine.

The amount of salt absorbed by the tubular cells depends on blood pressure and the concentration of certain hormones that affect the functioning of these cells. Thus, the kidneys regulate the balance of water and salt in the body. Conversely, the kidneys also affect blood pressure (for example, when blood pressure drops, more water and sodium are secreted into it).

The kidneys also produce a hormone called erythropoietin, which stimulates the production of red blood cells.

What renal failure can cause

Kidney damage can occur either suddenly, and as a result of the long-term disease process. If the kidneys are exposed to the damaging factor for a short time, acute renal failure (ONN) develops, characterized by a rapid increase in creatinine and a decrease in diuresis, and even complete anuria, often requiring renal replacement therapy. This condition can develop in a few hours to 7 days.

Nevertheless, acute failure may result in full recovery within a few months, and it mainly depends on the type of primary disease. However, if the kidney is damaged gradually through the long process of the disease (lasting at least three months) develop chronic kidney disease with the most severe forms: severe chronic kidney failure and end-stage renal disease, requiring dialysis.

Among the factors impairing kidney function are primarily the states of impaired blood flow, specific and non-specific inflammation and immunological factors and substances toxic to the kidneys, all processes can impair urinary tract patency and chronic diseases such as diabetes and hypertension.

Causes of acute renal failure

The factors responsible for acute kidney damage are divided into so-called prerenal, renal, and renal. The first, most common category includes conditions that disturb kidney blood flow, including:

• Decreased circulating the blood volume due to hemorrhage, dehydration, excessive diuresis, seepage into the body cavities or extensive burns and injuries;

• Heart disease characterized by a sudden decrease in stroke volume;

• States of the sudden increase in the volume of the vascular bed due to a vascular tone disorder (sepsis, antihypertensive, electrolyte disturbances, cirrhosis);

• Autoregulation of renal blood flow due to the use of non-steroidal anti-inflammatory drugs, cyclooxygenase inhibitors or angiotensin receptor blockers (drugs used in hypertension);

• Conditions of excessive blood viscosity, including hematologic malignancies

- Obstruction of the vessels supplying the kidneys due to a blood clot, embolism, aneurysm, external pressure, e.g., by a tumor or inflammation;

Renal factors that damage organ parenchyma include all glomerular inflammatory processes (autoimmune, allergic, viral, bacterial, idiopathic), systemic vasculitis, thrombotic microangiopathy, cholesterol embolism, malignant hypertension , autoimmune diseases including systemic lupus erythematosus and scleroderma systemic, damage to the renal parenchyma due to prolonged impaired blood supply, toxins - including contrast agents and drugs (including ciclosporin, cisplatin, some antibiotics, captopril, methotrexate, indinavir, acyclovir, ethylene glycol and methanol and - attention - popular non-steroidal drugs anti-inflammatory), as well as cancerous infiltrates.

Last but not least, the causes of ONN are conditions that cause obstruction of the urinary tract (also within the bladder) by urolithiasis, blood clots, fragments of damaged nipples, external pressure, e.g. by a cancerous tumor or in diseases of the prostate in men, interruption of the urinary tract or damage to the urethra.

Causes of chronic renal failure

In contrast to ONN, in this disease entity, kidney damage occurs gradually, primarily in the course of chronic diseases, such as:

- diabetes mellitus (diabetic nephropathy),

- hypertension (hypertensive nephropathy),

- glomerulonephritis and tubulointerstitial inflammatory processes,

- polycystic degeneration,

- systemic diseases, including sarcoidosis and amyloidosis

- less often long-term impaired blood flow or outflow of urine,

- plasma myeloma,

- HIV nephropathy

- genetically determined syndromes, e.g., Alport syndrome.

The Role of Sodium in the Body

Sodium is one of the elements necessary for the proper functioning of the body. He is primarily responsible for water and electrolyte management, but also has other functions. What are his other roles? Are there severe effects of excess and deficiency of sodium? How to introduce a diet that will allow us to reduce sodium intake?

The role of sodium in the body

Sodium has important functions in the body, and disturbances in its concentration can cause serious problems. The main tasks of this valuable element include:

- Maintaining the osmotic balance of the body in the extracellular fluids of the body - this means that it regulates the volume of water in the body and protects us from dehydration,

- Maintaining acid-base balance (together with potassium and chlorine),

- Involved in the conduction of nerve impulses - sodium is a potassium antagonist, and this element creates a concentration difference on both sides of the cell membrane, thus enabling the transmission of impulses. This process is responsible for the state of smooth muscle, skeletal and heart tension,

- Participation in the process of glucose and amino acid transport across cell membranes,

- Activating salivary amylase - a digestive enzyme present in saliva.

Normal sodium concentration in the body is 135-145 mmol /l, and its maintenance is responsible for the renin-angiotensin-aldosterone system. It is a complex hormonal-enzyme system that also regulates the volume of water in the body.

Potassium - role in the body

Potassium belongs to microelements and is an element that performs many essential functions. Thanks to potassium, our cells can transmit electrical impulses, but potassium also helps maintain adequate blood pressure and muscle tone.

Potassium, therefore, is an electrolyte, controls muscle function. It enables the generation of electrical impulses in the cells of our body, including in the cells of the heart muscles, i.e., it is responsible for each heartbeat. Potassium plays the same function in skeletal muscles.

Potassium is a sodium antagonist, and its opposite action consists of, among others, on reducing the volume of extracellular fluids, which helps to control the amount of water in the body. This role of potassium has also associated with the ability to maintain healthy blood pressure by lowering it.

Potassium is involved in the processes in which our cells synthesize proteins, which in turn are muscle building blocks. Thus, potassium is one of the factors that control muscle building and help maintain healthy muscle mass.

Potassium, being also a calcium antagonist, is responsible for proper muscle tone (so-called tonus) by raising their tone.

Also, potassium helps maintain acid-base balance, and thus maintain the homeostasis of the whole body.

Potassium and Our Health

If our body is functioning properly, balance is maintained between potassium and sodium. Disorders in the concentrations of these macroelements cause the occurrence of one of the most common and severe civilization diseases, i.e., hypertension and heart disease. Unlike sodium, low potassium levels promote these diseases.

People rarely suffer from potassium deficiency or bearing. This happens, however, in cases where the functioning of our body is disturbed.

Potassium deficiency, or hypokalemia, can occur when we use high blood pressure diuretics, in the case of prolonged vomiting or diarrhea, and with some kidney problems. Symptoms of hypokalemia are weak, flaccid muscles, arrhythmias, and a slight increase in blood pressure.

Hyperkalemia, which is too high in potassium, causes a dangerous arrhythmia. Hyperkalemia occurs when the kidneys are weak, infections are severe, and when you are taking some heart medicines.

Phosphorus - role in the body

Because as much as 85% of phosphorus is found in bones and teeth, it is necessary to maintain their proper structure. It also occurs in soft tissues and cell membranes, i.e., in the tissues of muscles, heart, and brain. It also plays an essential role in the process of growth and reconstruction or repair of damaged tissues. As one of the elements that take part in the processes occurring in the human body, phosphorus is also an energy transmitter. Thanks to this mineral, food is converted into energy that translates into muscle work.

Phosphorus also ensures the proper functioning of nerves and the brain and is involved in many chemical reactions and metabolic processes in our body. It maintains the overall vitality of the body. Also, it plays an important role in the work of the heart. For researchers, it is an essential carrier of genetic information because it is a component of DNA.

Diet for Kidney Failure: What to Eat and What to Avoid

In the diet for renal failure, it is necessary to control the intake of some nutrients such as sodium, phosphorus, potassium, and protein. In the most severe cases where the kidneys are no longer functioning well or in the case of dialysis, it is also necessary to control the number of fluids that are ingested daily. This includes water, juices, and soups.

When talking about kidney failure, it means that the kidneys' ability to filter waste from the blood and form urine is diminished, so it causes specific residues and minerals, such as those mentioned above, to accumulate in the blood and can cause serious consequences, this is due to the restriction of these nutrients in the diet.

So these individuals need to reduce the intake of proteins such as meats, fish, grains, and some types of fruits and legumes such as orange and kiwi. However, in the case of potassium-rich foods, some techniques can be used to reduce the amount of potassium in fruits and vegetables, such as peeling them before eating them.

Foods to be controlled

Renal insufficiency can be acute or chronic, so food restrictions in the diet vary according to the type of inadequacy and the stage in which the disease is found.

Ideally, in these situations, the individual should go to a nutritionist that specialized in the area to develop an individual nutritional plan based on the laboratory tests of the person, so the foods mentioned below should be consumed in moderation, since that the fact that they are ingested or not will depend on laboratory values:

1. Foods high in potassium

The kidneys of people with renal insufficiency have difficulty removing excess potassium from the blood, so those people need to control the intake of this mineral by avoiding abuse of them.

Potassium-rich foods are:

- Fruits: avocado, banana, coconut, fig, guava, kiwi, orange, papaya, passion fruit, tangerine, grape, raisins, plums, prune, melon, apricot, blackberries, and dates;

- Vegetables: potato, sweet potato, cassava, Creole celery, carrot, chard, beet, celery, cabbage, Brussel sprouts, radish, tomatoes, canned palm, spinach, turnip, and chicory;

- Legumes: beans, lentils, corn, peas, chickpea, soybeans, and beans;

- Whole grains: wheat, rice, and oats;

- Whole foods: biscuits, whole-wheat pasta, and breakfast cereals;

- Oleaginous: peanut, cashew, almonds, and hazelnuts;

- Industrialized products: chocolate, tomato sauce, meat, and chicken broth tablets;

- Drinks: coconut water, sports drinks, black tea, green tea, and matte tea;

- Seeds: sesame, and flaxseed;

- Paper or sugar cane guarapo ;

- Salt light

Too much potassium can cause muscle weakness, arrhythmias, and cardiac arrest, so the diet for chronic renal failure has to be individualized and accompanied by the doctor and the nutritionist, who will evaluate the appropriate amounts of nutrients that each person should ingest.

How to reduce potassium in the food

The following are some strategies that can help reduce the amount of potassium in fruits and vegetables:

- Peel fruits and vegetables;

- Cut and rinse food thoroughly;

- Place the plants to soak in water in the refrigerator for a day, before use;

- Place the food in a pot with water and boil for 10 minutes. Then drain the water and cook again with water and then prepare the food as desired.

Another important suggestion is to avoid the use of pressure cookers and microwaves to prepare meals since these techniques concentrate the potassium content in food by not allowing water to be changed.

2. Foods rich in phosphorus

Phosphorus-rich foods should also be consumed moderately by people with chronic renal failure to control kidney function. These foods are:

- Canned sins;

- Salted, smoked and sausage meats such as sausages;

- Bacon, bacon;

- Yolk;

- Milk and derivatives;

- Soy and derivatives;

- Beans, lentils, peas, corn;

- Oilseeds such as cashew, almonds, and peanuts;

- Seeds such as sesame and flaxseed;

- Coconut sweet;

- Beer, cola, and hot chocolate.

Symptoms of excess phosphorus are itchy body, hypertension, and mental confusion, and people with kidney failure should keep an eye on these signs.

3. Protein-rich foods

People with chronic renal failure need to control the consumption of proteins because, during their metabolism, toxic wastes are produced that accumulate in the blood, and cannot be eliminated. This is why it is essential to avoid excessive consumption of meat, fish, eggs, milk, and derivatives since they are foods rich in protein.

Ideally, a person with kidney failure should eat one small beef steak at lunch and dinner and one glass of milk or yogurt per day. However, this amount varies according to how the kidney function is, being more restrictive in those people in whom the kidney almost does not work.

4. Foods rich in salt and water

People with kidney failure also need to control salt intake, since the excess increases blood pressure and forces the kidney to work, further impairing the function of this organ. The same happens with the excess of liquids since these people produce little urine, and the excess of liquids ends up accumulating the organism, causing problems such as swelling and dizziness.

Therefore, the use of:

- Salt;

- Sauces such as ketchup, mayonnaise, aioli, among others;

- Tomato paste;

- Condiments such as cubes, soy sauce, and Worcestershire sauce;

- Canned food and frozen prepared food;

- Snacks, chips, and crackers with salt;

- Fast food;

- Powdered or canned soups.

A perfect option to avoid excess salt is to season foods with aromatic herbs such as parsley, garlic, and basil. The doctor or nutritionist will indicate the appropriate amount of salt and water allowed for each person individually.

How to choose snacks

Restrictions on the feeding of the renal patient can make it challenging to choose snacks. Therefore, the three most important recommendations for choosing healthy snacks are:

- Eat always cooked fruit (cook twice), never reusing cooking water, and it must be discarded;

- Restrict industrialized and processed foods that are generally rich in salt or sugars, preferring homemade preparations;

- Avoid the intake of protein foods in snacks.

Diet for acute renal failure

The diet for acute renal failure is usually performed at the hospital level, because it is a situation that occurs suddenly and is treated in the hospital, being carefully calculated by the nutritionist, and may even be necessary to use food through a route intravenously to administer the number of nutrients that the individual requires.

In general, renal function is usually restored, and the individual receives specific instructions on what they can eat to avoid the accumulation of toxins that are eliminated through the kidneys. Normally this diet is usually low in protein, potassium, salt, and phosphorus, as in chronic renal failure, until the function of the kidneys ultimately returns to normal.

Adapt to renal failure

Discovering that you have kidney failure can be a shock, even if you have known for a long time that your kidneys are not working well. But starting dialysis treatment doesn't have to say that the ones you enjoy are over. It may take a little time to adapt to your new routine, but you are not alone. Your doctors, nurses, and social workers can help you.

- Depression and anxiety

Depression is a feeling of sadness that extends for a long time. Anxiety is a feeling of nervousness that comes and goes.

It is normal for you to be nervous when you are going through significant changes in your life, mainly if these changes affect your health and well-being. When you start dialysis treatment, you may have to change your daily routine, your diet, and the type of activities you do. You will probably experience different feelings as you get used to this new lifestyle, such as sadness, fear, regret, and anger. You may not immediately understand what you are feeling, but you may notice that you feel strange.

Symptoms of depression are:

- Changes in sleeping patterns (sleeping too much or having trouble sleeping).

- Loss of interest in those activities you used to enjoy.

- Loss of appetite.

Some symptoms of anxiety are:

- Heart Rate Acceleration.

- Sweating.

- Breathe too fast.

- Difficulty thinking about anything except what worries you.

You must know that you are not alone. Most people have gone through what you are going through. Many people have felt like you. It is also essential that you know that you do not have to live with these feelings. Help is available. Talk to your social worker about the different ways to start feeling better. You may also find support groups useful.

- **Exercise**

Exercise is a perfect way to improve your health. Most people can and should exercise, even if they are undergoing dialysis treatment.

People who exercise regularly feel better, both physically and emotionally. Some benefits of exercise are:

- Mood improvement

- Improvement of heart and lung health

- Weightless

- Joint pain reduction

- Greater flexibility

Exercise does not have to be difficult or painful. If it hurts to perform a particular exercise, you shouldn't do it! There are many ways to exercise without experiencing pain or discomfort. Consider practicing low impact exercises.

These are exercises that do not cause too much tension in the joints.

- Hike

- Swimming

- riding a bicycle

- Yoga

- Pilates

- Use of elliptical machine

- Tai Chi

- Stretching

- Climbing stairs

You do not need to join a gym or buy expensive equipment to exercise.

You can walk in your neighborhood or the mall. Or you can practice yoga at home on the floor of your living room. Your doctor can help you design an exercise plan that is safe for you, and that suits your dialysis itinerary.

- **Job**

You may be able to continue working during your dialysis treatment. Working can help you feel happier and fulfilled. If you have health insurance through your work, staying in it will help you keep your insurance.

If you want or need to continue working during your dialysis treatment, talk to your doctor about your treatment options. Certain types of dialysis allow you to keep a more flexible schedule during the day.

For instance, if you choose night hemodialysis (at night), in the center or at home, you can perform your dialysis treatments at night, while you sleep. This is also possible with cyclist assisted continuous peritoneal dialysis (CCPD).

If you decide to continue working during your dialysis treatment, you must know your limits. You may feel tired or weak throughout the day. If you receive peritoneal dialysis treatment and make your exchanges, you must have a clean place in your work to do the exchanges. If you receive hemodialysis treatment, you should not lift heavy objects or put pressure on the arm of your vascular access.

Chapter Two: Everything You Need To Know About The Renal Diet

When you have kidney disease, you need to have a meal plan that includes a kidney diet. Taking notice of what you eat and drink will help you stay healthy. The facts in this section are for people who have kidney disease but do not receive dialysis treatment.

People are different, and we all have different nutritional needs. Talk to your renal dietitian (a person who is an expert in diet and nutrition for people with kidney disease) to find out which meal plan works best for you.

Ask your doctor to help you find a dietitian. Medicare policies and private insurance can help pay for appointments with dietitians.

Why Is It So Important To Follow A Meal Plan?

The things we were eating and drinking can affect your health. Maintaining a healthy weight and eating a balanced diet low in salt and fat can help control blood pressure. People with diabetes can help control blood sugar levels by choosing very carefully what to eat and drink. Controlling blood pressure and diabetes can help prevent kidney disease from getting worse.

A kidney diet helps prevent damage to the kidneys. The kidney diet limits certain foods and prevents the minerals of those foods from accumulating in the body.

Fundamentals of the Renal Diet

With all meal plans, including the renal diet, it is necessary to track the number of specific nutrients you consume, such as:

- Calories

- Protein

- Grease

- Carbohydrates

To make sure you're getting the right amount of these nutrients, you need to eat and drink the correct portion sizes. All the information you need to track your consumption is a "nutritional information" label.

Use the nutrition information section on meal labels to learn more about the foods you eat. The nutrition information will tell you how much protein, carbohydrates, fat, and sodium are in each serving of that meal. This can help you choose foods that are rich in the nutrients you need and low in the nutrients you should limit.

When you look at nutrition data, some key areas will give you the information you need:

- **Calorie**

Your body derives energy from the calories you eat and drink. Calories come from protein, carbohydrates, and fats in the diet. The amount of calories you need depends on your age, gender, body size, and activity level.

You can adjust your calorie intake according to your weight target. Some people limit the calories they eat. Others need to eat more calories.

- **Protein**

Protein is one of the essential components of the body. The body needs protein to grow, heal, and stay healthy. Too little protein can weaken skin, hair, and nails. But too much protein is a problem. To maintain health and improve mood. You may need to adjust the amount of protein consumed.

The number of protein you should consume depends on your body size, level of activity, and health problems. Some doctors recommend people with kidney disease to limit their protein or change their protein source. This is because a high-protein diet can hinder kidney function and cause damage.

- **Carbohydrates**

Carbohydrates are the simplest type of energy for your body to use. Some healthy sources of carbohydrates include fruits and vegetables. Unhealthy sources of carbohydrates include sugar, honey, candies, soda, and other sugary drinks.

Some carbohydrates are rich in potassium and phosphorus, which may be limited depending on your stage of kidney disease. You can also look at carbohydrate intake very carefully if you have diabetes. Your dietitian can help you know more about carbohydrates in your eating plan and how they can affect your blood sugar.

- **Grease**

You need some fat in your eating plan to stay up and healthy. Fat provides you energy and helps you to use some vitamins in food. But too much fat can result in weight gain and heart disease. Try to limit the fat in your eating plan and choose healthier fats when you can.

The healthiest fat or "good" fat is called unsaturated fat. Examples of unsaturated fats include:

- Olive oil

- Peanut oil

- Corn oil

Unsaturated fat can also help in reducing cholesterol. If you need to gain weight, try to eat unsaturated fats. If you need to lose weight, limit unsaturated fats in your eating plan. As always, moderation is the key. A lot of "good" fat can cause problems.

Saturated fat, also known as "bad" fat, can raise your cholesterol level and increase your risk for heart disease. Examples of saturated fats include:

- Butter

- Lard

- Shortening

- meats

Limit these fats in your eating plan. Choose healthy and unsaturated fats instead. Cutting the amount of fat in meats and removing the skin of chicken or turkey can also help limit saturated fat.

You should also avoid Tran's fats. This type of fat causes your "bad" cholesterol (LDL) to rise, and your "good" cholesterol to go down. When this happens, you may be more likely to get heart disease, which can cause kidney damage.

- **Sodium**

Sodium (salt) is a mineral in almost every meal. Excess sodium can lead to thirst, swelling, and an increase in blood pressure. This causes more kidney damage and hinders the work of the heart.

One of the best ways to stay healthy is to reduce your sodium intake. To limit your sodium intake in your meal plan:

- Never add salt to food while cooking or eating. Make an effort cooking with fresh herbs, lemon juice, or unsalted seeds.

- Choose between fresh or frozen vegetables instead of canned vegetables. If you use canned veggies, drain, and rinse to remove salt before cooking or eating.

- Keep away processed meats such as ham, bacon, sausage, sausage, and lunch.

- Eat fresh fruits and vegetables instead of pastries and other salty snacks.

- Keep away canned soups and high sodium frozen foods.

- Keep away pickles such as olives and pickles.

- Maximize spices with high sodium content such as soy sauce, grill, and tomato sauce (ketchup).

Important! Be careful with salt substitutes and "low-salt" foods. Many alternative salts are rich in potassium. If you have kidney disease, a lot of potassium is dangerous. Work with a dietitian to find foods that are low in sodium and potassium.

What Is The Difference Between Renal Diets?

When your kidneys are not functioning well as they should, wastes and fluids build up in your body. After a while, this waste and extra fluid can cause problems with the heart, bones, and other health problems. A renal diet eating plan can limit the number of certain minerals and fluids you consume. This can prevent waste and extra fluids from accumulating and causing problems.

How strict you need to be with your plan depends on your stage of kidney disease. In the early stages of kidney disease, there may be few or no limits on what you eat or drink. As time goes by and your kidney disease gets worse, your doctor may recommend that you limit the following:

- **Potassium**

Potassium is a mineral found in almost every meal. Your body needs some level of potassium for your muscles to work, but a lot of potassium can be dangerous in the body. When the kidneys are not functioning well, your potassium level may be too high or too low. Having too much or not enough potassium can cause muscle cramps, problems with the way your heartbeats, and muscle weakness.

If you have kidney disease, you can limit your potassium intake.

- **Match**

Phosphorus is a mineral found in almost every meal. Work with calcium and vitamin D to keep your bones healthy. Healthy kidneys maintain the correct level of phosphorus in your body. When your kidneys don't work well, phosphorus can accumulate. Excess phosphorus in your blood can lead to bone breakage easily.

- **Liquids**

Our body needs water to survive, but when you have kidney disease, you may not need it so much. This is because when the kidneys are damaged, they do not remove extra fluids as they should. Many liquids in your body can be dangerous. This can cause high blood pressure, swelling, and heart failure. Extra fluids that accumulate near your lungs can make it hard to breathe.

Special dietary concerns

Vitamins

Following a diet plan with a kidney diet may prevent your body from getting enough vitamins and minerals you need. To help you get the right levels of vitamins and minerals, your dietitian may suggest a supplement created for people with kidney disease.

Tumer or dietitians may also suggest a special type of vitamin D, folic acid, or iron pill to help prevent some of the typical side effects of kidney disease such as bone disease and anemia.

Regular use of many vitamins may not be healthy for you if you have kidney disease. They may contain much or too little vitamin.

After diabetic kidney meal

Should in case you have diabetes, you need to control blood sugar levels to prevent damage to the kidneys. A doctor or nutritionist can help you create a meal plan that enables you to control blood sugar levels while limiting sodium, phosphorus, potassium, and water. Diabetes educators can also learn to control blood sugar levels. Ask your doctor to introduce you to a diabetes educator in your area. Private insurance and Medicare can help you pay for reservations with diabetic educators.

Chapter Three: What Is Kidney Disease

The chronic renal failure or uremia is the inability of the kidneys to produce urine or fabricate low quality ("like water") since it not been removed enough toxic waste. Although some patients continue to urinate, most cannot. However, the important thing is not the quantity, but the composition or quality of the urine.

The kidneys are two "bean-shaped" organs, located in the dorsal wall of the body on the sides of the spine. They are brown, weigh about 150 grams each and are about 12 centimeters long, 6 centimeters wide, and 3 centimeters thick. In the upper part, each kidney has an endocrine gland attached (it produces vital substances inside the body) called the adrenal gland.

The kidneys are the "purifiers "where the blood is filtered and cleaned. They produce urine, which contains water, toxins, and salts that the blood has been collecting throughout the body, and that has to be eliminated. They also intervene in other activities such as reproduction, because they make sex hormones; regulate the amount of phosphorus and calcium in the bones; they control the tension in the blood vessels, and manufacture substances that are involved in blood clotting.

Renal insufficiency appears when only 5 percent of the total kidney or nephron filters work. The basic unit of the kidney is the nephron, of which there are about 1 million in each organ. Each nephron is formed by a component that acts as a filter, the glomerulus, and a transport system, the tubule.

Some of the blood that reaches the kidneys is filtered by the glomerulus and passes through the tubules, where various excretion and reabsorption processes occur that give rise to the urine that is eventually removed.

The renal blood flow (RBF or amount of blood reaching the kidney per minute) is approximately adult 1.1 liters per minute. Of the 0.6 liters of plasma that enter the glomerulus through the arterioles, 20 percent are filtered, an operation called renal glomerular filtration.

The renal glomerular filtrate is, therefore, the volume of plasma filtered by the kidneys per unit of time. The amount of filtered plasma per day is 135 to 160 liters. To prevent fluid loss, between 98 percent and 99 percent of the renal glomerular filtration rate is reabsorbed by the tubules, resulting in the amount of urine removed resulting from between one and two liters per day.

When a kidney disorder occurs, it means that one or more of the renal functions are altered. But not all functions are altered in the same proportion; for example, if two thirds of the nephrons cease to function, significant changes may not occur because the remaining nephrons adapt; Likewise, changes in hormonal production may go unnoticed, and then the calculation of renal glomerular filtration is the only way to detect the decrease in the number of nephrons that continue to function.

Cause of Kidney Disease

Renal failure occurs when a disease or other health condition impairs kidney function, causing damage to the kidneys, which tend to get worse over several months and even years. Diseases and conditions that usually cause chronic kidney disease include:

- Type 1 and 2 Diabetes

- Hypertension

- Glomerulonephritis, which is inflammation of the glomeruli, functional units of the kidneys where blood filtration occurs.

- Interstitial Nephritis

- Polycystic Kidney Disease And Other Congenital Diseases That Affect Kidneys.

- Prolonged urinary tract obstruction due to specific conditions such as prostatic hyperplasia, kidney stones, and some cancers.

- Vesicoureteral reflux

- Recurrent renal infection also called pyelonephritis.

- Autoimmune Diseases

- Kidney injury or trauma

- Overuse of painkillers and other medicines

- Use of some toxic chemicals

- Kidney Artery Problems

- Reflux Nephropathy

Chronic renal failure leads to an accumulation of fluid and waste in the body. This disease affects most body systems and functions, including red blood cell production, blood pressure control, vitamin D levels, and bone health.

Risk factors

Factors that are likely to increase a person's risk of developing chronic renal failure include:

- Diabetes

- Hypertension

- Heart diseases

- Smoke

- Obesity

- High cholesterol

- Be African American, Native American, or Asian American

- Have a family history of kidney disease

- 65 years or older

Symptoms of Chronic Kidney Failure

Chronic kidney disease slowly worsens over time. In the early stages, it may be asymptomatic. Loss of function usually takes months to occur. It can be so slow that symptoms do not appear until kidney function is less than one-tenth of normal. That is, when the person realizes, he is usually already with the functioning of the kidneys completely compromised.

Early symptoms of chronic renal failure usually also frequently occur in other diseases, and maybe the only signs of renal failure until it is advanced.

Symptoms may include:

- General malaise and fatigue

- Generalized itching (itching) and dry skin

- Headaches

- Unintentional Weight Loss

- Loss of appetite

- Nausea

Other symptoms that may appear, especially when kidney function worsens include:

- Abnormally light or dark skin.

- Bone pain.

- Drowsiness and confusion.

- Difficulty concentrating and reasoning.

- Numbness in hands, feet and other body areas.

- Muscle spasms or cramps.

- Bad breath.

- Easy bruising, bleeding or bloody stools.

- Excessive thirst.

- Frequent hiccups.

- Low level of sexual interest and impotence.

- Interruption of the menstrual period (amenorrhea).

- Sleep disorders such as insomnia, restless legs syndrome, and sleep apnea.

- Swelling of hands and legs (edema).

- Vomiting, usually in the morning.

Chapter Four: Steps To Control Chronic Kidney Failure

Seek treatment for hypertension

T*he pressure is now considered the leading cause of chronic renal failure. According to nephrologist Nestor Scho, professor at Unifesp, the increase in blood pressure damages the blood vessels of the kidneys and may cause hypertensive nephropathy. "This way, the organ becomes overloaded, and little by little loses its filtering capacity," he explains. Taking care of hypertension is essential even when it is not the cause of chronic renal failure, as it becomes even more important in the advanced stage of the disease.*

Control of diabetes

"Diabetes is the second leading cause of chronic renal failure," says nephrologist Lucio Roberto Requião Moura of Hospital Israelita Albert Einstein. This is because the disease triggers the so-called diabetic nephropathy, a change in kidney vessels that leads to a protein loss in the urine. Also, diabetes favors atherosclerosis, the formation of plaque fat in the arteries that hinders the filtration work of the kidneys. Over time, more and more toxic substances are trapped in the body, which can lead to death. One way to detect the problem, therefore, is to do urine tests to find out if the protein is being eliminated. Those already diagnosed with diabetes need to be more aware of their kidney health.

Watch the weight

Overweight people (Discover their ideal weight) have a higher risk of developing hypertension and diabetes, which is reason enough not to let the scale hand rise, says nephrologist Lucio. Added to this is the fact that obesity alters the way blood reaches the kidneys by the influence of certain hormones, overloading the organ. Moreso, being overweight is a risk factor for high cholesterol and triglycerides.

Adapt your diet

When it comes to food, analyzing the underlying disease that triggered kidney failure is critical. If it is diabetes, for example, the diet should be the right diet for those with diabetes. If it is hypertension, then there should be reduced salt intake. "However, in general, it is recommended that the patient avoid excessive protein intake, especially of animal origin, which gives rise to toxic elements in the body that would make the kidneys work harder," explains nephrologist Nestor. In specific cases of insufficiency yet, there may be retention of potassium in the body. Patients with this problem need to prepare food in a way that causes them to release some of this nutrient. For example, vegetables need to be cooked.

Inquire about medications

The self-medication is dangerous even for healthy people. For those with kidney failure, however, use without proper medical evaluation can accelerate kidney deterioration. "The most dangerous are non- hormonal anti-inflammatory drugs," warns nephrologist Lucio. Therefore, explain your problem at the beginning of every medical appointment to avoid aggravating the disease.

Way to drink alcohol

Although no studies are proving the isolated relationship between alcohol intake and chronic renal failure, alcohol abuse compromises the functioning of the body as a whole. Thus, it is recommended to handle consumption. If you are having a drink, however, nephrologist Nestor advises opting for wine. "It contains antioxidants that can help eliminate concentrated toxins in the body," he says

Put out the cigarette.

"Cigarettes are responsible for worsening blood pressure levels and are still involved with hormonal changes that worsen kidney function," explains nephrologist Lucio. Also, smoking triggers a vasoconstriction effect, decreasing the volume of blood filtered by the kidneys. In this case, there is no moderation option. The patient must end the addiction.

Practice exercises

The last recommended care for chronic kidney failure sufferers is regular exercise. "It prevents diabetes, hypertension, obesity, among other problems, and improves circulation and kidney function," says nephrologist Nestor. According to him, any activity is already better than physical inactivity, but it is always recommended to seek training that pleases the patient so that he does not feel discouraged over time.

Chapter Five

Renal Diet Recipes

Liver of heifer and its onion compote

INGREDIENTS

- 1 slice of organic heifer liver
- 2 small onions
- 1 apple Canada
- tablespoon of olive oil
- 1 lemon
- 1 slice of cinnamon
- Salt pepper

DIRECTIONS

1. Peel and slice the onions. Make them return in half of the olive oil until they become translucent. Salt and pepper them. Cover and cook on very low heat for 30 minutes. Watch for cooking, add a little water if necessary.

2. Wash the lemon under running water, wipe it and squeeze it.

3. Wash the apple, peel it, and remove the fibrous core and seeds. Cut it into cubes. Lemon it to avoid blackening, place in a small saucepan with cinnamon and 2 tablespoons of water. Cook covered over low heat for 20 minutes. At the end of cooking, crush it in the coarse compote.

4. Cut the liver into strips and cook for 2 to 3 minutes in the pan with the remaining olive oil. Once cooked, mix it with the onion compote.

5. Enjoy it immediately, accompanied by the applesauce.

Nutritional interest

Thanks to the liver, this dish is very rich in iron and zinc, easily assimilated, trace elements essential for the proper functioning of the immune system. It may be particularly recommended for young children, regulated women, and endurance athletes, who often lack iron.

In case of excess cholesterol, do not consume more than one shot per week.

Palette of pork and its vegetables

INGREDIENTS

- 1 pallet of bone-in pork of 1 kilo
- 100 g of smoked diced bacon
- 1/4 green cabbage
- 300 g of carrots
- 200 g of turnips
- 400 g of firm-fleshed potatoes type BF 15
- 2 onions
- 2 cloves
- 1 bouquet garni
- 1 tablet of organic vegetable broth
- Salt pepper

DIRECTIONS

1.   Place the bacon in a saute pan and sauté over medium heat, stirring. Add the palette and use the fat rendered to brown the meat, about 5 minutes on each side. Add a peeled onion and chopped, also brown. Add 1/2 liter of water, the bouquet garni, and the second onion stuck cloves and the crumbled broth.

2.   Wash the piece of cabbage, remove the outer leaves too hard, and its core. Dip it in a pan of boiling salted water and let it whiten for 10 minutes. Drain it and cut it into strips. Add it to the sauté pan with the palette, salt, and pepper it, continue cooking for 15 minutes.

3.   Wash and peel carrots, turnips, and potatoes. Cut them into slices. Add the carrots and turnips in the pan, salt, and pepper. Continue cooking for 10 minutes. Add the potatoes and cook for 20 minutes. Rectify the seasoning, remove the bouquet garni and onion pique clove.

Nutritional interest

This complete dish simultaneously brings functional meat proteins, fiber, and vitamins from vegetables, energy carbohydrates from potatoes. Low fat; it is suitable for overweight (450 kcal per serving). For a balanced meal, add milk and seasonal fruit.

Exotic Fruit Verrines

INGREDIENTS

- 2 kiwis

- 1 mango

- 1/2 grenade

- 1/4 liter of semi-skimmed milk

- 2 eggs

- 25 g of sugar

- 1 vanilla pod

- 2 half-sheets of gelatin or 1/2 teaspoon of agar agar

DIRECTION

1.　　Wash the vanilla pod, slice it in half, and place it in a saucepan with the milk. Heat and stop the fire just before boiling. Let the vanilla steep in the milk.

2.　　Position the gelatin in a bowl of cold water.

3.　　Separate the whites and egg yolks. Whip the yolks with the sugar. Add the cooled and filtered milk. Pour everything into the saucepan and cook on low heat, continually stirring until the cream thickens. Add drained half-leaves of gelatin or agar-agar, wait for their complete dissolution to cut the fire. Divide the custard into four glasses and refrigerate for at least 2 hours.

4.　　Wash the fruits under running water and sponge them out. Peel the kiwis and mango and cut them into cubes. Collect the grains from the pomegranate. Mix these fruits gently and divide them into the glasses. Enjoy it immediately.

Nutritional interest

Thanks to exotic fruits, these verrines are rich in antioxidant vitamins: beta-carotene, vitamins B9, and C, which help the body defend itself against infections.
To balance your menu, consume a verrine at the end of a meal with vegetables, meat, fish or legumes, and starchy foods.

Chickpea Salad

INGREDIENTS

- 150 g of chickpeas

- 1 onion

- 1 clove

- 1 clove of garlic

- 1 bouquet garni

- 200 g of celery-branch

- 1 lemon
- 5 tablespoons of olive oil
- 1 tip of curry
- 1 tablespoon of chopped chives
- Salt pepper

DIRECTION

1. Position the chickpeas in a large bowl filled with cold water and let them soak for 12 hours.

2. Peel the onion and garlic. Drain the chickpeas. Place them in a casserole with 1/2 liter of cold water, the bouquet garni, and the onion stuck clove, the clove of garlic, some grains of pepper. Cover, cook for 2 hours.

3. Wash the celery, detach its branches from the bulb, remove the top of the leaves, detail it in the sticks.

4. Wash the lemon and squeeze its juice — mix 2 tablespoons with the olive oil and the curry.

5. Drain the chickpeas well. Mix with celery. Add salt and pepper. Season with the olive oil vinaigrette and add the chives.

Nutritional interest

- This salad, rich in fiber and protein (chickpeas) is very satiating and has a low glycemic index. It can be especially recommended in case of diabetes. Calorie intake reasonable 250 kcal per serving. It is suitable for overweight.

- The consumption of pulses is recommended at least twice a week to increase vegetable protein and reduce animal protein.

Roquefort pear toast

INGREDIENTS

- 8 slices of walnut bread (120 g)
- 1 jar of 100 g of white cheese with 3% fat
- 60 g of Roquefort cheese
- 2 ripe Williams or Guyot pears
- 1 lemon
- 4 nuts

DIRECTIONS

1. Toast the slices of bread.

2. Remove the nuts from their shells.

3. Mix the cottage cheese and Roquefort cheese. Spread toast with this mixture.

4. Wash the lemon, sponge it, and squeeze its juice.

5. Wash the pears, peel them, remove their central part and their pips, divide them into tiny dice. Lemon immediately to prevent the pears from turning black.

6. Spread the pears over the toasts. Add a walnut kernel per toast.

Nutritional interest

- Made from walnut bread, Roquefort pear toasts provide 25% of the recommended daily intake of omega 3 essential fats, which are beneficial for cardiovascular prevention. They are rich in fiber (bread, pear, nuts), satiating, and regulating the transit.

- Spread with lean fresh cheese with 3% fat and a small amount of Roquefort, they are suitable for hypercholesterolemia.

- Whether you eat them as a starter or as an appetizer, you can balance your meal by moderating starchy foods and preparing vegetables.

Shortbread with jam

INGREDIENTS

- 100 g of wheat flour type 55
- 50 g of butter or margarine rich in omega 3 not lightened
- 50 g of sugar
- 1 egg
- 120 g of strawberry or apricot jam, homemade if possible
- 2 tablespoons of icing sugar
- 1 large star-shaped cookie cutter
- 1 round-shaped cookie cutter 1.5 cm in diameter

DIRECTIONS

1. Separate the whites from the egg yolk.

2. In a bowl, mix the flour, sugar, and butter until you have a texture of sand. Add the egg yolk to mix the dough ball. Let the dough rest in the refrigerator for at least 30 minutes.

3. Preheat the oven to 180 ° C. Arrange a sheet of baking paper on a baking sheet.

4. Spread the dough. Cut star-shaped shortbread. In half of these shortbreads, cut a small circle of dough in the middle.

5.   Arrange the shortbread on the plate and bake for 15 minutes.

6.   Let the shortbread a little cool. Cover each shortbread with jam and sprinkle each shortbread with icing sugar. Arrange the shortbreads pierced over jammed biscuits.

Nutritional interest

•   Made with flour and jam, these biscuits are rich in carbohydrates and energy. They have their place at the end of a meal without starch or snack after a light lunch. They can also be used as a snack, in recovery after a sports training.

•   Low in fat, they are suitable for hypercholesterolemia.

Skewers of seitan

INGREDIENTS

•   1 block of seitan 240 g

•   1 lemon

•   3 tablespoons of sesame oil

•   2 onions

•   1 clove of garlic

•   1 tablespoon of acacia honey

•   1 tablespoon of paprika

•   200 g of cherry tomatoes

•   100 g of Paris mushrooms

•   2 tablespoons of sesame seeds

•   Salt pepper

DIRECTIONS

1.   Wash the lemon under running water, sponge it, and squeeze it.

2.   Peel the onions, slice them. Peel and slice the clove of garlic.

3.   Cut the seitan into cubes.

4.   Mix honey and lemon juice, add oil and paprika, salt, and pepper. Arrange the seitan, onions, and garlic in a dish and sprinkle with the marinade. Allow in the refrigerator for at least 1 hour.

5.   Wash the tomatoes and mushrooms, sponge them out. Cut the mushrooms into strips.

6.   Make skewers by alternating seitan cubes with onion rings, cherry tomatoes, and mushroom slices. Filter the marinade.

7.   Cook the kebabs on a pan in their marinade for 2 to 30 minutes on each side over medium heat. Drain them and roll them in the sesame seeds. Iron for one minute in the pan, just time to lightly brown the sesame seeds.

Nutritional interest

These skewers provide as much protein as a small steak, the quality of which can be optimized by combining legume proteins, such as lentils. With a reasonable energy intake of 280 kcal, they are suitable for overweight.

Bean salad to shell

INGREDIENTS

- 150 g of shelling beans
- 30 g of pasta, farfalle type
- 150 g of fresh green beans

- 200 g of tomatoes
- 1 carrot
- 1 bouquet garni
- 4 tablespoons of olive oil
- 2 tablespoons of balsamic vinegar
- 1/2 teaspoon of mustard
- 1 shallot
- 2 teaspoons of chopped parsley
- 1 teaspoon of chopped basil
- Salt pepper

DIRECTIONS

1. Shell the beans. Position them in a large saucepan and cover them completely with cold water. Add the bouquet garni, cover the pan. Let it simmer for 35 minutes.

2. Wash the green beans and mop them up. Cut in half, salt, and steam for 15 minutes.

3. Cook the pasta the time indicated on the package.

4. Peel and chop the shallot.

5. Prepare the vinaigrette with oil, vinegar, mustard, salt, and pepper. Add the shallot.

6. Wash tomatoes and carrot under running water. Rind off and grate the carrot, cut the tomatoes into wedges.

7. In a salad bowl, combine the shelling beans and the drained pasta, the green beans, the tomatoes, the carrot, and the herbs. Add the vinaigrette and mix gently. Correct the seasoning if necessary.

Nutritional interest

This salad is rich in fiber and antioxidants: vitamin E, vitamin C, lycopene (tomatoes), beta-carotene (carrot). It combines the complementary proteins of beans to shelling and pasta. By doubling the proportions, you will get a balanced vegetarian main course.

Raspberry tartlets without gluten

INGREDIENTS

- 100 g of rice flour

- 30 g of almond powder

- 30 g of butter or margarine rich in omega 3 not lightened

- 90 g of sugar

- 2 eggs

- 20 g of cornflower

- 25 cl of semi-skimmed milk

- 1 vanilla pod

- 500 g of raspberries

- 1 tablespoon of icing sugar

DIRECTIONS

1.   Heat the milk until boiling. Cut the fire. Split the vanilla pod in half and let it steep in the milk.

2.   Mix the rice flour with the almond powder and 60 g of sugar. Add the melted butter and work the dough with a fork until you get a sandy texture. Combine the dough with one beaten egg and refrigerate for at least 30 minutes.

3.   Separate the white and yellow from the remaining egg. Whip the yolk with 30 g of sugar. Add the cornflower, then the

milk, previously filtered, very gradually. Cook this cream over low heat, constantly stirring until thickened (about 3 minutes).

4.   Preheat the oven to 180 ° C. Spread the pie dough and divide it into four lightly greased tart pans. Cover each tart with parchment paper and dried vegetables — Cook the tarts for 25 minutes.

5.   Wash the raspberries under a stream of running water. Sponge them carefully and remove their peduncles.

6.   Wait until the tartlets are cold to garnish with pastry cream and raspberries. Sprinkle with icing sugar.

Nutritional interest

Made from rice flour and corn, this tart is suitable for gluten intolerance. Thanks to raspberries, it is a good source of fiber and vitamin C. Energetic; it has its place at the end of a meal without starchy foods.

Quiche with ratatouille

INGREDIENTS

- 250g of flour

- 125 g of butter or margarine rich in omega 3 not lightened

- 2 zucchini

- 1 eggplant

- 3 tomatoes

- 1 yellow pepper

- 1 onion

- 2 tablespoons of olive oil

- 1 bouquet garni

- 4 eggs
- 100 g of grated Emmental cheese
- Salt pepper

DIRECTIONS

1.   In a small salad bowl, mix the flour and butter until you have a texture of sand. Add a little salt water to combine the ball of dough. Let stand in the refrigerator for at least 30 minutes.

2.   Peel and slice the onion. Wash the vegetables. Peel the zucchini and cut into slices. Cut the eggplant into cubes. Remove the peduncle, seeds and whitish fibrous parts of pepper, cut into strips.

3.   Fry the onion with the olive oil in a frying pan. Add pepper, zucchini, and eggplant, brown while stirring. Add the tomatoes, the bouquet garni, salt, and pepper. Cover; simmer on low heat for 20-30 minutes. At the end of cooking, discover to let evaporate the water of constitution of vegetables.

4.   Preheat the oven to 200-210 ° C. Spread the dough and place it in a pie dish. Cover with parchment paper and dried vegetables — Cook for 20 minutes.

5.   Mix the well-reduced ratatouille with the eggs and Emmental cheese. Pour this mixture onto the pie shell, free of parchment paper. Finish cooking in the oven for 15 minutes.

Nutritional interest

The ratatouille quiche is a complete balanced dish, which can be supplemented with dairy and fresh fruit.

Zucchini or shrimp verrines

INGREDIENTS

- 2 zucchini

- 2 shallots

- 2 tablespoons of olive oil

- 1/4 teaspoon of curry

- 100 g of shelled shrimp

- 1 bunch of chervil

- Salt pepper

DIRECTION

1. Peel and mince the shallots.

2. Wash the zucchini, sponge them, peel them, and cut them in small dice.

3. Place the oil in a pan with the curry. Add the shallots and zucchini to make them come back. Add salt and pepper. Cover, cook for 15-20 minutes over low heat. At the end of cooking, if necessary, evaporate the vegetable water.

4. Divide the zucchini fondue into 4 verrines. Add the shrimp on top and decorate with chervil sprigs.

Nutritional interest

Made from ingredients from the Mediterranean diet, this verrine provides multiple antioxidants (vitamins C and E, beta-carotene, polyphenols, and selenium) to protect the health. Very low fat and low in calories (100 kcal per serving), it is particularly suitable for hypercholesterolemia or overweight.

Homemade sauerkraut

INGREDIENTS

- 1 white cabbage, preferably organic
- 2 teaspoons of salt
- 1 teaspoon of juniper berries
- 1 teaspoon of peppercorns
- 6 bay leaves
- 2 glass jars of 1 liter with a screw lid

DIRECTION

1. Wash the jars and their lid thoroughly.

2. Put away the outer leaves and the core of the cabbage. Cut it into skinny strips.

3. In each jar, alternate layers of cabbage, each with salt, juniper berries, peppercorns, and bay leaves. Pack well.

4. If there is a bit of room at the top of the jar, add water that has been boiled and chilled. Close the jars without screwing them in completely.

5. Leave the jars at room temperature for 2 days, so that the cabbage can ferment. Then, screw them thoroughly and place them in the refrigerator for 1 month before eating. You can keep them for up to 6 months. Once started, consume them within 48 hours.

Nutritional interest

- Preparing homemade sauerkraut helps to consume raw. And so, to enjoy more of its vitamins (C and B9 in particular) and natural lactic ferments at the origin of its obtaining. Some of these ferments reach the colon alive and contribute to the functional diversity of the microbiota (intestinal flora), favorable to health.

- Namely: 100 g of sauerkraut provides 100% of the daily need for vitamin K, a contribution that must be taken into account by people on anticoagulant therapy.

Homemade yogurts with a pressure cooker

INGREDIENTS

- 90cl of semi-skimmed UHT milk
- 1 jar of plain yogurt with commercial whole-milk
- 4 tablespoons of skimmed milk powder
- 1 organic orange
- 1 cooking thermometer

DIRECTIONS

1. Wash the orange under running water, sponge it with absorbent paper and recover its zest.

2. Place the milk and orange zest in a saucepan, heat to a boil. Then, turn off the heat and let the zest infuse until the milk temperature drops to 45 ° C (check with the thermometer).

3. During this time, fill the pressure cooker with water for one third. Close the lid and put it on the fire. Leave several

minutes under pressure. Then, cut the fire and let the steam escape.

4.   Sift the milk through the sieve to remove the orange zest. Whisk it with yogurt and milk powder. Divide into eight glass yogurt jars.

5.   Discard the boiling water from the pressure cooker. Place the pots in the basket of the casserole and enclose them immediately in the still very hot casserole. Let it ferment at room temperature for 4 - 5 hours. Then place the yogurt in the refrigerator.

Nutritional interest

Yogurt makes it possible to take advantage of the good proteins and the calcium of the milk, even in case of intolerance to lactose (sugar of cow, goat, and sheep milk), that its lactic ferments have the capacity to digest. It can be called probiotic, because its regular consumption contributes to the development, within the microbiota (intestinal flora), of bacteria considered as beneficial to health.

Omelet with chicken livers

INGREDIENTS

- 6 eggs
- 150 g of chicken livers
- 2 shallots
- 3 tablespoons of olive oil

- 1 tsp of chopped parsley, 1 teaspoon of chopped chives, 1 tsp of chopped tarragon

- Salt pepper

DIRECTIONS

1. Pare and cut in 4 the chicken livers. Peel and mince the shallots.

2. Fry the chicken livers in the olive oil and cook for 3 to 4 minutes. Then, reserve them and sweat the shallots over a relatively soft fire. Mix them with the livers and reserve.

3. Beat the eggs, salt and pepper them. Cook them in a sloppy omelet. Spread over the chicken livers and herbs.

4. Fold the omelet and slide it onto a serving dish.

Nutritional interest

- Poultry liver omelet provides good protein that is effective for growing children, as well as maintaining muscle mass in adults. It is a good source of vitamin D: 2g per serving, or 40% of the recommended daily intake.

- Its reasonable caloric intake (225 kcal) allows us to consume it in case of overweight.

- To know: this recipe is not recommended for pregnant women and children under three years because of the very high vitamin A content of chicken livers.

CHEESECAKE

INGREDIENTS

- 350 g of 3% fat (3% fat) white cheese enriched with vitamin D (Calin + type)

- 2 eggs

- 35 g of Maïzena ®
- 60 g of sugar
- 1 teaspoon of bitter almond extract
- 1 tablespoon of flaked almonds
- Salt

DIRECTIONS

1. Preheat the oven to 170 ° C. Garnish a mold to run out of baking paper.

2. Separate the yolks and whites from the eggs. Climb these in very firm snow with a pinch of salt.

3. Mix the Maïzena® gradually with the cottage cheese. Then add the egg yolks, the sugar, then the almond extract. When the preparation is homogeneous, gently add the egg whites.

4. Pour the dough into the mold and bake for 40 to 45 minutes. Check the cooking by pricking the cake with a knife tip. Wait until it has cooled down to remove the baking paper.

5. Pass the almonds quickly in a non-stick frying pan for browning. Decorate the cake.

Nutritional interest

The cottage cheesecake provides good protein (cottage cheese, egg), as well as energy carbohydrates (sugar, Maizena). Made from white cheese enriched with calcium and vitamin D, it provides respectively 25 and 100% of the recommended daily intake to an adult in these micronutrients. It may be particularly recommended for growing teenagers and seniors for the prevention of osteoporosis.

Pear and walnut

INGREDIENTS

- 1 beautiful pear
- 80 g of butter
- 1/2 teaspoon of vanilla extract
- 2 eggs
- 100 g of sugar
- 50 g of chestnut flour
- 50 g of wheat flour type 55
- 1/2 sachet of yeast
- 80 g of unsweetened cocoa powder
- 14 nuts
- 2 teaspoons of icing sugar

DIRECTIONS

1.   Preheat the oven to 180 - 200 ° C. Lightly grease a non-stick mold with an oiled brush.

2.   Wash the pear, peel it, remove its central part and its seeds, cut it in big quarters. Put it in the pan with 20 g of butter and vanilla. Remove it from the fire as soon as it begins to caramelize. Arrange it at the bottom of the mold.

3.   Schell nuts.

4.   Separate the whites from the egg yolks. Beat the egg whites with a pinch of salt.

5.   Mix the egg yolks with the sugar. Add the remaining 60 g of butter. Gradually add the two flours with the yeast, then the

cocoa powder, and finally 12 nuts. Carefully incorporate the whites into the snow.

6.   Pour the mix into the pan over the pear and bake for 25 minutes at 180 ° C. Check the cooking with a knife tip (the dough does not stick when the cake is cooked).

7.   Unmount the pound. Sprinkle with icing sugar and decorate with the remaining 2 nuts.